200 Low-Carb Recipes

RECISES

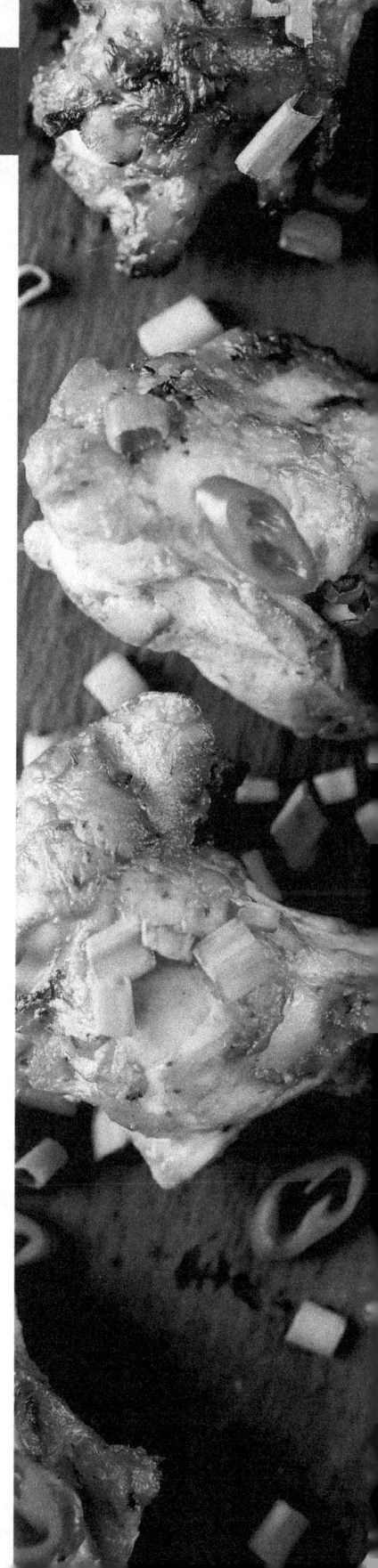

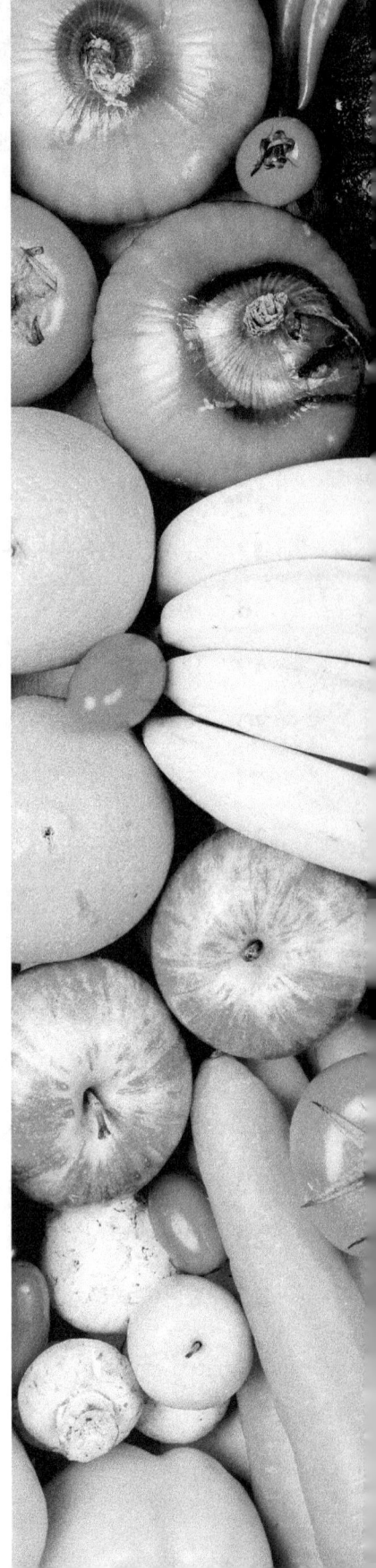

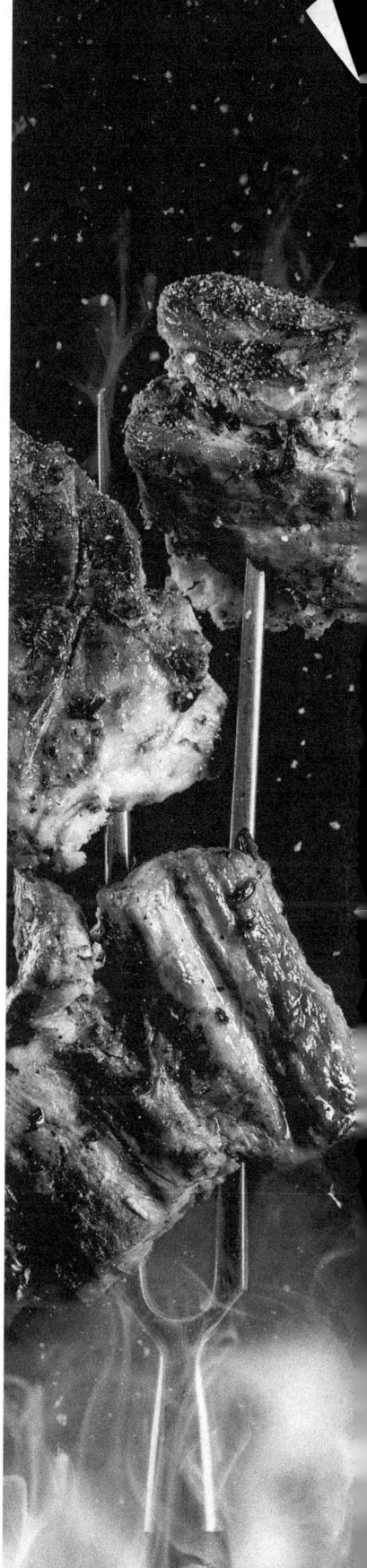

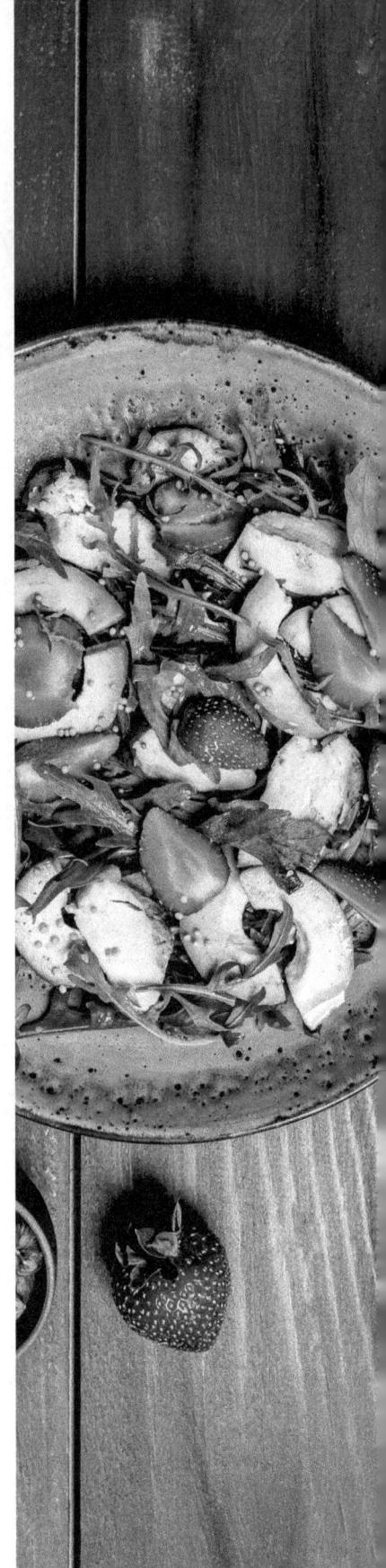

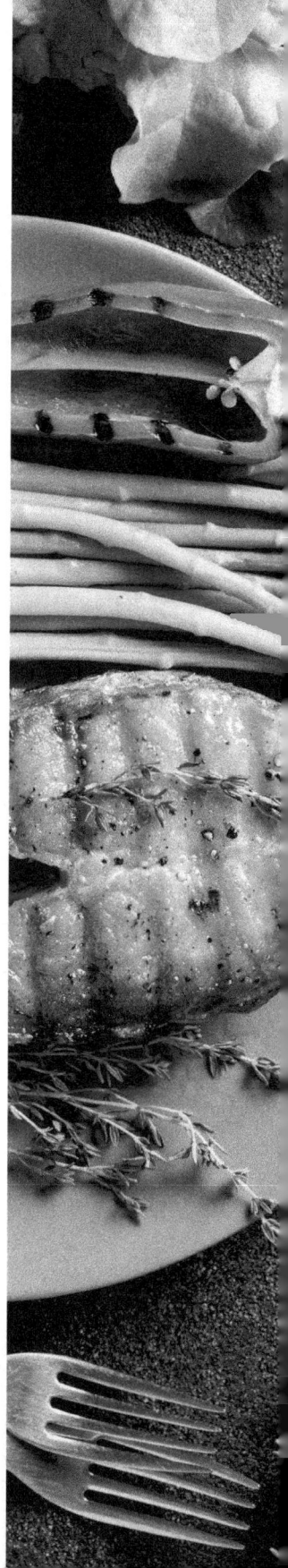

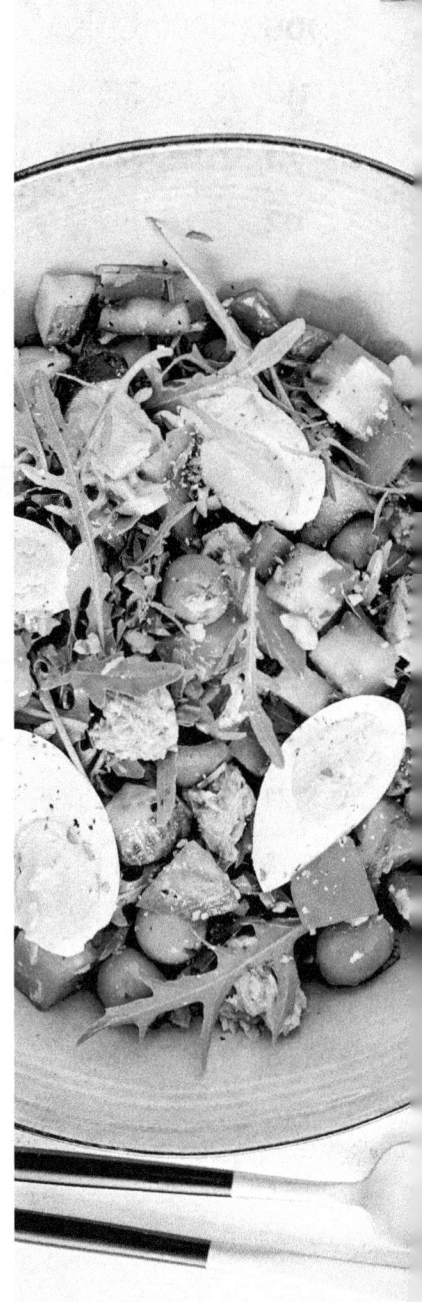

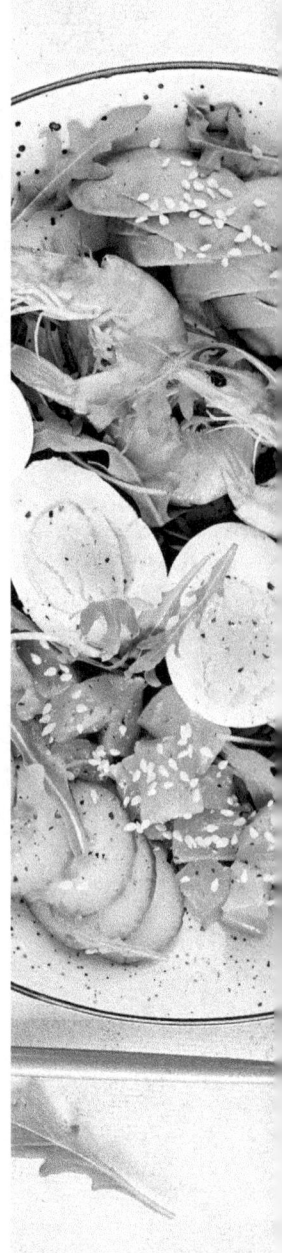

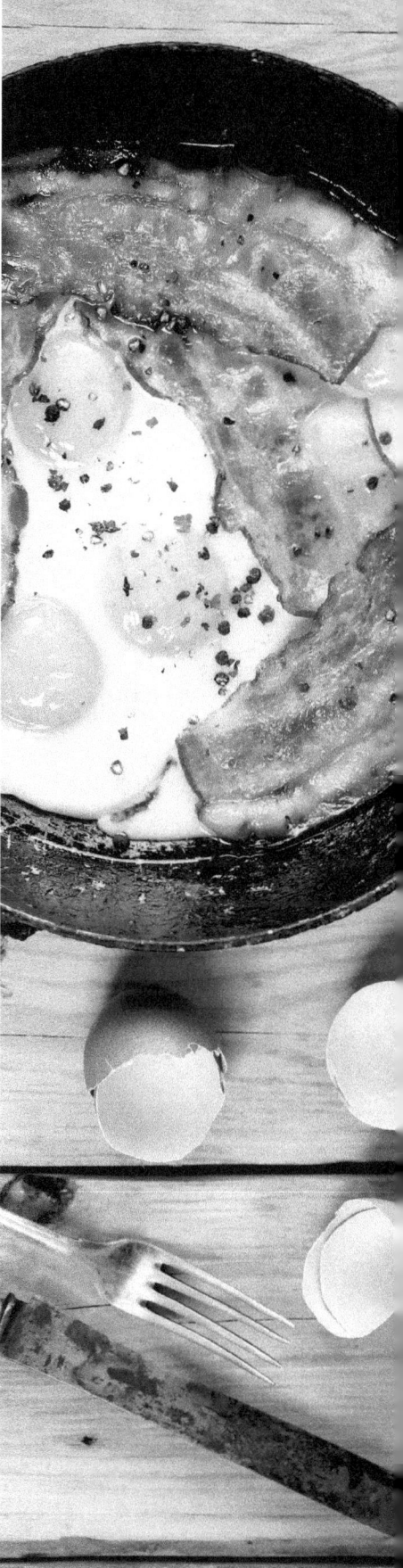

GRILLED VEGETABLE SOUP

SERVES FOR
6 PEOPLE

INGREDIENTS

1/4 cup shredded basil leaves
1/2 tsp. dried oregano
1 tsp. olive oil
1 red onion, peeled and cut into 1/2-inch-thick slices
1 yellow bell pepper, and quartered lengthwise
1 clove garlic
1 Tbsp. red-wine vinegar
2 red bell peppers, and quartered lengthwise
1/2 lb. zucchini, trimmed and quartered lengthwise
3 large vine-ripened tomatoes
Salt & freshly ground black pepper

STEPS

1. Prepare a grill or preheat the broiler. Grill bell peppers, skin-side toward the flame, for about 10 minutes. Place in a paper bag and set aside for 15 minutes.

2. Meanwhile, brush zucchini and onion slices with oil and grill, about 6 minutes. Chop coarsely and set aside.

3. Peel the peppers. Coarsely chop the yellow pepper and set it aside with the reserved zucchini and onions. Place the red peppers in a blender, along with tomatoes, oregano, and garlic; puree until smooth. Transfer to a bowl and stir in 1 cup water, basil, vinegar, and the reserved chopped vegetables. Season with salt and pepper. Cover and refrigerate until cool.

4. Serve!

NUTRITION FACTS

Calories: 56 |Fat: 1 g|Carbohydrates: 11 g|Sodium: 12 mg|Protein: 2 g| Cholesterol: 0 mg

CUMIN-CRUSTED SEA BASS

SERVES FOR
4 PEOPLE

INGREDIENTS

1/4 tsp. freshly ground black pepper
1/2 tsp. salt
1/2 Tbsp. olive oil
1 Tbsp. cumin seeds
1 lb. sea bass fillets, skinned and cut into
4 pieces
1-1/2 Tbsp. chopped fresh parsley
Lemon wedges

STEPS

1. Preheat oven to 350 degrees F.

2. In a dry skillet, toast cumin seeds over medium heat, stirring, for 4 minutes.

3. Transfer to a bowl to cool.

4. With a spice grinder and pestle, grind cumin seeds, salt, and pepper into a fine powder. Rub spice mixture on both sides of bass.

5. In an ovenproof skillet, heat oil over medium heat. Add bass fillets and cook until browned, for 6 minutes.

6. Transfer skillet to oven and bake until fish is opaque in the center, for about 8 minutes.

7. Garnish with parsley and serve immediately, with lemon wedges!

NUTRITION FACTS

Calories: 130 |Fat: 4 g|Carbohydrates: 1 g|Fiber: 0 g| Sodium 345 mg | Protein: 21 g| Cholesterol: 47 mg

FILLET OF SOLE WITH SPINACH

SERVES FOR
4 PEOPLE

INGREDIENTS

1 lb. sole fillets
2 cloves garlic, minced
4 small plum tomatoes, sliced
12 cups spinach, trimmed
Salt & freshly ground black pepper

STEPS

1. Preheat oven to 425 degrees F. Prepares 4 pieces of parchment paper for papillotes. Put spinach, with water still clinging to its leaves, into a pot. Cover; steam the spinach over medium heat, stirring occasionally, for 6 minutes. Drain; when cool enough to handle, press out excess liquid.

2. Chop and place in a bowl. Stir in garlic. Season with salt and pepper. Place one-quarter of the spinach mixture in the center of one-half of each opened paper heart. Lay a sole fillet over the spinach and arrange tomato slices over the sole. Season with salt and pepper. Seal the packages and place them on a baking sheet. Bake for 13 minutes.

3. Transfer the packages to individual plates.

4. Serve!

NUTRITION FACTS

Calories: 156 |Fat: 2 g|Carbohydrates: 9 g|Protein: 27g| Sodium: 231 mg|Cholesterol: 55 mg

MUSTARD-CRUSTED SALMON

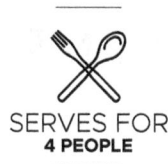

INGREDIENTS

1/4 cup reduced-fat sour cream
1-1/4 pounds center-cut salmon fillets, cut into 4 portions
2 tablespoons coarse-grained mustard
2 teaspoons fresh lemon juice
4 lemon wedges
Salt & freshly ground black pepper to taste

STEPS

1. Line a metal pan with foil, then lightly oil. Preheat broiler.

2. Place salmon pieces, skin-side down, in a prepared pan. Season with salt and pepper. In a bowl, combine mustard, sour cream, and lemon juice. Spread evenly over salmon.

3. Broil salmon, 5 inches from the heat source, for 13 minutes.

4. Serve with lemon wedges.

NUTRITION FACTS

Calories: 255 |Fat: 10 g|Carbohydrates: 1 g|Sodium: 90 mg|Protein: 29 g|Cholesterol: 83 mg| Protein: 29 g

SHRIMP WITH BROCCOLI

SERVES FOR
4 PEOPLE

INGREDIENTS

1/2 tsp. cornstarch
1/2 tsp. crushed red pepper
1 Tbsp. olive oil
1 Tbsp. minced garlic
1 lb. large shrimp, peeled and deveined
2/3 cup water
2/3 cup bottled clam juice
2 Tbsp. chopped fresh basil
4 cups fresh broccoli florets
Lemon juice
Freshly ground black pepper
Lemon wedges
Salt

STEPS

1. In a nonstick skillet, heat 1/2 Tbsp. oil over medium heat. Add 1/2 Tbsp. garlic and crushed red pepper; cook, stirring, for about 1 minute. Add shrimp and season with salt. Sauté for about 4 minutes. Transfer to a bowl; set aside.

2. Add remaining 1/2 Tbsp. oil to skillet. Add broccoli and season with salt. Sauté until bright green, about 1 minute. Add water, cover, and cook for about 5 minutes. Transfer broccoli to the bowl with shrimp.

3. In another bowl, combine clam juice, remaining 1/2 Tbsp. garlic and cornstarch; stir until smooth. Add to skillet and cook, stirring, over medium-high heat, until thickened, for 4 minutes. Stir in basil and season with lemon juice and pepper. Add reserved shrimp and broccoli and heat through.

4. Serve with lemon wedges.

NUTRITION FACTS

Calories: 185 |Fat: 6 g|Carbohydrate: 7 g|Protein: 26 g|Fiber: 3 g| Sodium: 285 mg|Cholesterol: 175 mg

SWORDFISH KEBABS

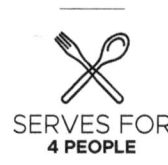

SERVES FOR
4 PEOPLE

INGREDIENTS

1/4 tsp. freshly ground black pepper
1/2 tsp. salt
1 Tbsp. olive oil
1 Tbsp. chopped fresh rosemary
1 lb. swordfish steaks, cut into 1 1/4-inch cube
1 small zucchini, sliced into 1/4-inch-thick ovals
2 Tbsp. lemon juice

STEPS

1. Prepare a grill. If using wooden skewers, soak eight 10-inch skewers in water for 15 minutes.

2. In a shallow dish, stir together olive oil, lemon juice, rosemary, salt, and pepper. Add swordfish and stir to coat well. Cover with plastic wrap and marinate in the refrigerator for 20minutes.

3. Thread skewers alternately with pieces of swordfish and zucchini.

4. Grill the kebabs on a lightly oiled grill rack for about 5 minutes per side.

5. Serve!

NUTRITION FACTS

Calories: 177 |Fat: 8 g|Carbohydrates: 2 g|Sodium: 370 mg| Protein: 23 g|Cholesterol: 44 mg

BRAISED GREEN BEANS & TOMATOES

INGREDIENTS

1/4 tsp. crushed red pepper
1 Tbsp. fennel seeds, crushed
1 lb. green beans, trimmed
2 tsp. olive oil
4 cloves garlic, thinly sliced
8 ripe tomatoes, peeled, seeded and chopped
Salt & freshly ground black pepper

STEPS

1. In a saucepan of boiling salted water, cook green beans until just tender, for 5 minutes. Drain and refresh with cold water.

2. In a Dutch oven, heat oil over medium heat. Add garlic and cook, stirring, until fragrant, about 40 seconds. Add fennel seeds and crushed red pepper; cook, stirring, for 40 seconds more. Add green beans and tomatoes. Cover and cook, stirring often, until tomatoes form a sauce and beans are soft, about 25 minutes. Season with salt and pepper.

3. Serve!

NUTRITION FACTS

Calories: 80 |Fat: 2 g|Carbohydrates: 14 g|Fiber: 2 g|Sodium: 20 mg|Protein: 3 g|Cholesterol: 0 mg

BROCCOLI WITH CARAMELIZED SHALLOTS

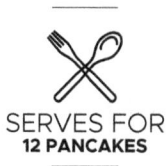

SERVES FOR
12 PANCAKES

INGREDIENTS

1 cup sliced shallots, thinly sliced
1 bunch broccoli, cut into florets
1 1/2 tsp. olive oil
2 Tbsp. walnut pieces
Salt & freshly ground black pepper

STEPS

1. Preheat oven to 450 degrees F. Place walnuts on a pie plate and toast in the oven for 5 minutes. Transfer to a bowl and set aside.

2. In a nonstick skillet, heat oil over low heat. Add shallots and cook, stirring often, for about 12 minutes. Season with salt and pepper; set aside in the skillet.

3. Meanwhile, cook broccoli in boiling salted water for 5 minutes. Drain the broccoli and add it to the shallots in the skillet and toss to combine.

4. Transfer to a serving bowl and garnish with the toasted walnuts.

5. Serve!

NUTRITION FACTS

Calories: 113 |Fat: 4 g|Carbohydrates: 16 g|Protein: 7 g|Sodium: 51 mg|Cholesterol: 0 mg

SAUTÉED CHERRY TOMATOES WITH CHIVES

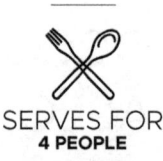

SERVES FOR
4 PEOPLE

INGREDIENTS

2 tsp. olive oil
2 Tbsp. chopped fresh chives
2 pts. cherry tomatoes
Salt & freshly ground black pepper to taste

STEPS

1. In a skillet, heat oil over medium heat. Add tomatoes and sauté, for 4 minutes. Remove from heat, toss with chives, and season with salt and pepper.
2. Serve!

NUTRITION FACTS

Calories: 52 |Fat: 3 g|Carbohydrate: 7 g|Sodium: 12 mg|Protein: 1 g|Cholesterol: 0 mg

SAVOY CABBAGE WITH PEPPERS

INGREDIENTS

1/4 cup defatted reduced-sodium chicken broth
1/4cup chopped bottled roasted red peppers
1/2 teaspoon caraway seeds
1/2 teaspoon mustard seeds
1 jalapeño pepper, seeded and finely chopped
2 teaspoons vegetable oil, preferably canola oil
4 cups thinly sliced Savoy cabbage
Salt & freshly ground black pepper to taste

STEPS

1. In a nonstick skillet, heat oil over medium heat. Add caraway and mustard seeds and cook, stirring, for 1 minute. Stir in jalapeños and cabbage, cook, stirring, for 1 minute.

2. Stir in chicken broth and cover the pan tightly. Reduce heat to low and simmer, for 6 minutes. Stir in red peppers and season with salt and pepper.

3. Serve!

NUTRITION FACTS

Calories: 51 |Fat: 3 g|Carbohydrates: 6 g|Sodium: 48 mg|Protein: 2 g|Cholesterol: 0 mg

GREEN BEANS WITH SESAME

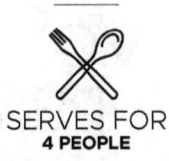

INGREDIENTS

1 teaspoon olive oil
1 pound green beans, trimmed
2 teaspoons sesame seeds
Salt & freshly ground black pepper

STEPS

1. Preheat oven to 425 degrees F. On a baking sheet with sides, toss beans with oil, then spread the beans out in a single layer. Roast the beans for 15 minutes, stirring once.

2. In a dry skillet over medium heat, stir sesame seeds until fragrant and toasted, about 1 minute. Crush the seeds lightly and toss with the beans. Season with salt and pepper.

3. Serve!

NUTRITION FACTS

Calories: 60 |Fat: 2 g|Carbohydrates: 9 g|Sodium: 4 mg|Protein: 2 g|Cholesterol: 0 mg

WILTED SPINACH WITH GARLIC

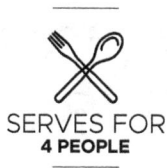

SERVES FOR
4 PEOPLE

INGREDIENTS

1 Tbsp. olive oil
1 clove garlic, finely chopped
1 lb. spinach, washed and stemmed
Salt & freshly ground black pepper

STEPS

1. Heat oil in a skillet over medium heat. Add garlic and stir, about 40 seconds. Add the spinach and toss until just wilted, for about 5 minutes. Season with salt and pepper.

2. Serve!

NUTRITION FACTS

Calories: 56 |Fat: 4 g|Carbohydrates: 4 g|Sodium: 90 mg|Protein: 3 g|Cholesterol: 0 mg

HALIBUT WITH HERBS & CAPERS

SERVES FOR
4 PEOPLE

INGREDIENTS

1/8 teaspoon freshly ground pepper
1/4 cup chopped onion
1/4 cup fresh flat-leaf parsley
1 pound halibut fillet, cut into 4 portions
1 tablespoon fresh cilantro leaves
1 tablespoon fresh lemon juice
1 tablespoon chopped pitted green olives
1 clove garlic, minced
2 teaspoons drained capers, rinsed
2 tablespoons extra-virgin olive oil
2 teaspoons freshly grated lemon zest

STEPS

1. Place onion, cilantro, parsley, lemon zest, lemon juice, capers, olives, garlic, and pepper in a food processor; pulse several times to chop. Add oil and process, until pesto-like paste forms. Sprinkle halibut with the herb paste. Cover and refrigerate for 25 minutes.

2. Preheat oven to 450 degrees F. Coat a baking dish with cooking spray. Arrange the halibut in the dish and spoon any extra herb mixture on top. Bake, uncovered, for 20 minutes.

3. Serve immediately!

NUTRITION FACTS

Calories: 199 |Fat: 10 g|Carbohydrates: 2 g|Fiber: 1g| Sodium:125 mg|Protein: 24 g|Cholesterol: 36 mg

CHICKEN BREASTS

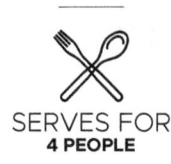

SERVES FOR
4 PEOPLE

INGREDIENTS

1 tablespoon dark brown sugar
2 tablespoons dried jerk seasoning
2 teaspoons reduced-sodium soy sauce
2 teaspoons canola oil
3 tablespoons lime juice
4 boneless, skinless chicken breast halves, trimmed
6 scallions, trimmed and coarsely chopped

STEPS

1. Combine scallions, lime juice, jerk seasoning, soy sauce, sugar, and oil in a blender; pulse to a coarse paste. Spread the paste all over the chicken. Cover and marinate in the refrigerator for at least 30-40 minutes.

2. Lightly oil broiler rack and set it 5 inches from the heat source; preheat broiler.

3. Scrape most of the paste from the chicken and discard. Broil chicken, turning once, until juices run clear, for about 15 minutes. Let stand for 2 minutes before slicing.

4. Serve!

NUTRITION FACTS

Calories: 192 |Fat: 6 g|Carbohydrates: 7 g|Fiber: 1 g|Sodium: 450 mg|Protein: 28 g|Cholesterol: 73 mg

CHEESY FRITTATA

SERVES FOR
2 PEOPLE

INGREDIENTS

1/4 cup fat-free evaporated milk
1/2 cup sliced onion
1/2 cup sliced red bell pepper
1/2 cup sliced zucchini
1/2 cup liquid egg substitute
1/2 cup 1% cottage cheese
1 tablespoon chopped fresh basil
2 teaspoons Smart Balance spread
2 small plum tomatoes, diced
3/4 ounce shredded reduced-fat
Monterey Jack cheese
Pinch freshly ground black pepper

STEPS

1. Coat an ovenproof skillet with cooking spray and place over medium heat until hot.

2. Melt the spread in the skillet. Add the bell pepper, onion, and zucchini and sauté over medium-low heat, for about 3 minutes. Add the tomatoes, basil, and black pepper to the skillet and stir to combine. Cook, for 2 minutes, and remove from the heat.

3. Preheat the broiler. In a blender, combine the egg substitute, cottage cheese, and milk and process until smooth. Pour the egg mixture over the vegetables. Cover and cook on medium-low heat until the bottom is set and the top is still slightly wet. Transfer the skillet to the broiler and broil until the top is set, for about 3 minutes. Sprinkle with the cheese and broil until the cheese melts.

4. Serve!

NUTRITION FACTS

Calories: 231 |Fat: 10 g|Carbohydrates: 16 g|Fiber: 2 g|Sodium: 480 mg|Protein: 21 g|Cholesterol: 15 mg

ASPARAGUS AND MUSHROOM OMELET

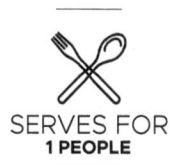

SERVES FOR
1 PEOPLE

INGREDIENTS

1/4 cup sliced white mushrooms
1/4 cup shredded reduced-fat
mozzarella cheese
2 eggs
2 tablespoons water
3 stalks fresh asparagus

STEPS

1. Boil 1" of water in a skillet. Add the asparagus and cook, uncovered, just until tender.

2. Meanwhile, in a bowl, whisk together the eggs and water until the whites and the yolks completely blended.

3. Coat a 10" nonstick skillet with cooking spray. Heat the skillet over medium heat until just hot enough. Pour in the egg mixture. It should set immediately.

4. With an inverted pancake turner, lift the edges as the mixture begins to set to allow the uncooked the portion to flow underneath.

5. When the top is set, fill one-half of the omelet with the asparagus, mushrooms, and cheese.

6. With the pancake turner, fold the omelet in half over the filling. Slide onto a serving plate.

7. Serve immediately!

NUTRITION FACTS

Calories: 238 |Fat: 15 g|Carbohydrates: 5 g|Protein: 21 g|Sodium: 260 mg|Fiber: 1 g|Cholesterol: 440 mg

VEGETABLE QUICHE

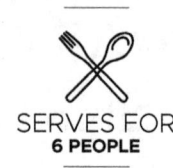

SERVES FOR
6 PEOPLE

INGREDIENTS

1/4 cup diced green bell peppers
1/4 cup diced onions
3 drops hot-pepper sauce
3/4 cup liquid egg substitute
3/4 cup shredded reduced-fat cheese
10 ounces frozen chopped spinach

STEPS

1. Place a microwave the spinach for 3 minutes on high. Drain the excess liquid.

2. Line a 12-cup muffin pan with foil baking cups. Spray the cups with cooking spray.

3. Combine the egg substitute, peppers, onions, cheese, and spinach in a bowl. Mix well. Divide evenly among the muffin cups. Bake at 375 degrees F for 18 minutes.

4. Quiche cups can be frozen and reheated in the microwave.

5. Serve!

NUTRITION FACTS

Calories: 77 |Fat: 3 g|Carbohydrates: 3 g|Fiber: 2 g|Protein: 9 g|Sodium: 160 mg|Cholesterol: 10 mg

CHICKEN PISTACHIO SALAD

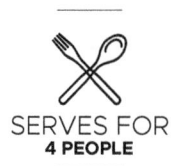

SERVES FOR
4 PEOPLE

INGREDIENTS

Dressing
1 teaspoon grated sweet white onion
1 large ripe avocado, pitted and peeled
1 tablespoon water
3 tablespoons extra-virgin olive oil
3 tablespoons fresh lime juice

Salad
1/2 cup shelled pistachio nuts, finely ground
1/2 + 1/4 teaspoon salt
1/2 teaspoon + 1 pinch freshly ground black pepper
1/2 cup diced sweet white onion
1 head romaine lettuce
2 tablespoons extra-virgin olive oil
4 boneless, skinless chicken breast halves

STEPS

1. To make the dressing: Puree the avocado, oil, onion, lime juice, and water in a blender.

2. To make the salad: Preheat the oven to 400 degrees F. Mix the nuts on a pie plate with 1/2 teaspoon salt and 1/2 teaspoon pepper. Press the chicken into the pistachio nuts. Heat 1 tablespoon of the oil in a skillet and cook the coated breasts, for 3 minutes for the side. Place the breasts in a baking dish and bake for 13 minutes.

3. Heat the remaining tablespoon of oil in a nonstick skillet over high heat. Add the diced onion, 1/4 teaspoon salt, and a pinch of pepper. Cook until the onion is browned.

4. Line 4 serving plates with lettuce. Slice the chicken breasts and arrange 1 breast on top of the lettuce on each plate. Garnish with the dressing.

5. Serve!

NUTRITION FACTS

Calories: 481 |Fat: 34 g|Carbohydrates: 13 g|Fiber: 5 g|Protein: 33 g|Sodium: 520 mg|Cholesterol: 70 mg

CRAB SALAD

SERVES FOR
2 PEOPLE

INGREDIENTS

1/4 cup crumbled blue cheese
1/4 cup olive oil vinaigrette
6 ounces crabmeat, drained
1 cup diced ripe tomatoes, halved
2 tablespoons cholesterol-free bacon bits
6 cups romaine lettuce, torn into bite-size pieces

STEPS

1. Arrange the lettuce on a serving platter. Arrange the crab meat, blue cheese, tomatoes, and bacon bits in rows over the lettuce.

2. Right before serving, drizzle some dressing evenly over the salad and toss well.

3. Transfer to the 2 chilled plates.

4. Serve!

NUTRITION FACTS

Calories: 267 |Fat: 13 g|Carbohydrates: 12 g|Fiber: 4 g|Sodium: 1012 mg|Protein: 27 g|Cholesterol: 95 mg

MIXED VEGETABLES WITH CRABMEAT SALAD

INGREDIENTS

1/2 cup sliced water chestnuts
1/2 cup julienne-sliced red bell pepper
2 cups torn curly endive
2 cups loosely packed watercress leaves
2 cups torn fresh spinach
2 cups torn red leaf cabbage
12 ounces crabmeat, fresh
Joe s mustard sauce

STEPS

1. Combine the endive, spinach, cabbage, watercress, water chestnuts, and pepper in a bowl.

2. Toss well. Add the crabmeat.

3. Divide onto 4 serving plates. Garnish with Joe's Mustard Sauce.

4. Serve!

NUTRITION FACTS

Calories: 123 |Fat: 1 g|Carbohydrates: 9 g|Fiber: 4 g|Sodium: 338 mg|Protein: 20 g|Cholesetrol: 76 mg

CHICKEN WITH BALSAMIC VINEGAR

SERVES FOR
6 PEOPLE

INGREDIENTS

1/4 cup balsamic vinegar
1/2 teaspoon freshly ground black pepper
1/2 teaspoon salt
1 1/2 teaspoons fresh rosemary leaves, minced
2 cloves garlic, minced
2 tablespoons extra-virgin olive oil
5 tablespoons white wine
6 boneless, skinless chicken breast halves

STEPS

1. Rinse the chicken and pat dry. Combine the garlic, rosemary, pepper, and salt in a small bowl and mix well. Place the chicken in a bowl. Sprinkle with the oil, and rub with the spice mixture. Cover and refrigerate overnight.

2. Preheat the oven to 425 degrees F. Spray a heavy roasting pan with cooking spray. Place the chicken in the pan and bake for 13 minutes. Turn the chicken over. If the drippings begin to stick to the pan, stir 4 tablespoons white wine.

3. Bake for about 12 minutes. If the pan is dry, stir in another 1–2 tablespoons of white wine to loosen the drippings. Sprinkle the vinegar over the chicken in the pan.

4. Transfer the chicken to plates. Stir the liquid in the pan and drizzle over the chicken.

5. Serve!

NUTRITION FACTS

Calories: 183 |Fat: 6 g|Carbohydrates: 4 g|Fiber: 0 g|Protein: 26 g|Sodium: 270 mg|Cholesterol: 65 mg

GINGERED CHICKEN BREAST

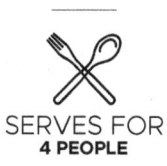

INGREDIENTS

1/2 teaspoon freshly ground black pepper
1 tablespoon fresh lemon juice
1 1/2 teaspoons grated fresh ginger
2 cloves garlic
4 boneless, skinless chicken breast halves

STEPS

1. Combine the ginger, lemon juice, pepper, and garlic in a bowl.

2. Place the chicken breasts in a deep bowl. Pour the ginger mixture over the breasts, turning once to coat both sides. Cover, and refrigerate for 1 hour.

3. Sprinkle a nonstick skillet with cooking spray. Heat the skillet on medium until hot. Add the chicken, cook, turning once, for about 10 minutes.

4. Serve!

NUTRITION FACTS

Calories: 129 |Fat: 1 g|Carbohydrates: 1 g|Fiber: 0 g|Protein: 26 g|Sodium: 75 mg|Cholesterol: 65 mg

GRILLED STEAK WITH TOMATO RELISH

INGREDIENTS

1/4 cup chopped fresh basil
1 medium onion, chopped
1 clove garlic, minced
2 sirloin steaks
2 medium pear-shaped tomatoes, halved lengthwise
2 tablespoons extra-virgin olive oil
Pinch salt
Pinch freshly ground black pepper
Basil sprigs

STEPS

1. Place the steak on a lightly greased grill above a solid bed of medium-hot coals. Cook, turning as needed for about 15 minutes.

2. Meanwhile, place the tomatoes on the grill, cut sides up, and brush them lightly with 1 tablespoon of the oil. When the tomatoes are browned on the bottom, about 3 minutes, turn them over and continue to cook until soft when pressed for about 3 more minutes. While the tomatoes are grilling, combine the remaining 1 tablespoon of oil, the onion, and garlic in a frying pan, set on the stove over medium-high heat. Cook, stirring often for about 8 minutes. Stir in the basil. When the tomatoes are soft, stir them into the onion mixture, then set the pan aside on a cooler area of the grill.

3. When the steak is done, place it on a board with a well. Spoon the tomato relish alongside the steak. Season with salt and pepper and garnish with basil sprigs.

4. To serve, cut the meat into thin slices. Combine the accumulated meat juices with the tomato relish.

NUTRITION FACTS

Calories: 366 |Fat: 22 g|Carbohydrates: 11 g|Fiber: 3 g|Protein: 31 g|Sodium: 70 mg|Cholesterol: 85 mg

GRILLED SALMON WITH ROSEMARY

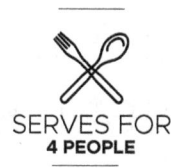

SERVES FOR
4 PEOPLE

INGREDIENTS

1/4 teaspoon salt
1 pound salmon
2 teaspoons extra-virgin olive oil
2 teaspoons fresh lemon juice
2 cloves garlic, minced
2 teaspoons fresh rosemary leaves,
chopped, crushed
Fresh rosemary sprigs
Capers
Pinch freshly ground black pepper

STEPS

1. Cut the fish into 4 equal-size portions. Combine in a bowl the lemon juice, olive oil, garlic, salt, pepper, and rosemary in a bowl. Brush the mixture onto the fish. To grill, arrange the fish on a grill rack.

2. Grill over medium-hot coals until the fish flakes easily for about 7 minutes.

3. To serve, garnish the fish with capers, and rosemary sprigs.

NUTRITION FACTS

Calories: 231 |Fat: 15 g|Carbohydrates: 1 g|Protein: 23 g|Sodium: 213 mg|Cholesterol: 67 mg

COD WITH GREEN ONION AND GINGER SAUCE

SERVES FOR
2 PEOPLE

INGREDIENTS

1/4 cup finely chopped green onion
1/3 cup dry sherry
1 teaspoon freshly grated ginger
1 teaspoon finely chopped garlic
2 teaspoons sesame oil
2 cod fillets
3 tablespoons low-sodium soy sauce

STEPS

1. Preheat the oven to 425 degrees F.
   Mix the sherry, sesame oil, soy sauce,
   ginger, onion, and garlic in a bowl.

2. Place the fish fillets in an ovenproof
   casserole dish. Sprinkle the marinade
   over the fish and bake for about 10
   minutes.

3. Serve!

NUTRITION FACTS

Calories: 242 |Fat: 6 g|Carbohydrates: 3 g|Fiber: 1 g|Protein: 35 g|Sodium: 1154 mg|Cholesterol: 45 mg

SHRIMP ROLLED WITH BACON

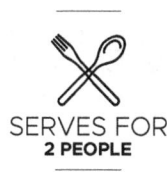

INGREDIENTS

10 slices bacon
20 large shrimp, peeled and deveined
Olive Oil

STEPS

1. Preheat grill for medium heat.

2. Wrap shrimp in bacon, and secure with toothpicks.

3. Lightly grease a grill with the oil and arrange shrimp on the grill.

4. Cook for 5 minutes, turning once.

5. Serve!

NUTRITION FACTS

Calories: 853 |Fat: 81 g|Carbohydrates: 0.8 g|Sodium: 1126 mg|fiber: 0 g|Cholesterol: 200 mg

OVEN-ROASTED VEGETABLES

INGREDIENTS

1/2 teaspoon freshly ground black pepper
1 medium red bell pepper, cut into bite-size pieces
1 medium yellow bell pepper, cut into bite-size pieces
1 medium zucchini, cut into bite-size pieces
1 medium summer squash, cut into bite-size pieces
1 pound fresh asparagus, cut into bite-size pieces
1 red onion
1 teaspoon salt
3 tablespoons extra-virgin olive oil

STEPS

1. Heat the oven to 425 degrees F. Place the squash, zucchini, peppers, asparagus, and onion in aroasting pan. Sprinkle with olive oil, salt, and pepper to mix and coat. Spread in a single layer in the pan. Roast for 40 minutes, stirring occasionally.

2. Serve!

NUTRITION FACTS

Calories: 170 |Fat: 11 g|Carbohydrates: 15 g|Fiber: 5 g|Protein: 5 g|Sodium: 586 mg|Cholesterol: 0 mg

ROASTED EGGPLANT AND PEPPERS

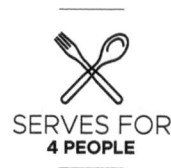

INGREDIENTS

1/4 cup extra-virgin olive oil
1 green bell pepper, cut in thick strips
1 onion, sliced
1 eggplant, peeled, halved, and sliced
2 red bell peppers, cut in thick strips
Fresh basil

STEPS

1. Preheat the oven to 375 degrees F. Place the peppers, eggplant, and onion in a nonstick baking dish.

2. Sprinkle with the oil. Bake in the oven for 18 minutes tossing regularly.

3. Arrange the vegetables on a serving dish and garnish them with fresh basil.

4. Serve!

NUTRITION FACTS

Calories: 193 |Fat: 14 g|Carbohydrates: 16 g|Fiber: 5 g|Protein: 2 g|Sodium: 5 mg|Cholesterol: 0 mg

SPINACH-STUFFED MUSHROOMS

INGREDIENTS

1/8 teaspoon salt
1/2 cup water
1 tablespoon extra-virgin olive oil
8 large mushrooms
10 ounces frozen chopped spinach

STEPS

1. In a saucepan, bring 1/2 cup water to a boil. Add the spinach and salt. Cover, and cook according to package directions. Wash the mushrooms. Remove the stems, trim off the ends, then chop the stems.

2. Heat the olive oil in a skillet. Add the chopped mushroom stems. Sauté until golden, for 4 minutes. Remove from the pan. Add the mushroom caps to the skillet and sauté for 5 minutes. Remove the mushroom caps to a heatproof serving platter.

3. Drain the spinach. Stir in the sautéed chopped mushrooms.

4. Spoon the spinach mixture into the cups and serve immediately.

NUTRITION FACTS

Calories: 33 |Fat: 2 g|Carbohydrates: 3 g|Fiber: 2 g|Protein: 2 g|Sodium: 74 mg|Cholesterol: 0 mg

STEWED TOMATOES AND ONIONS

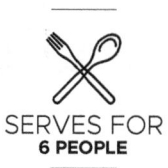

INGREDIENTS

1/8 teaspoon freshly ground black pepper
1/4 cup thinly sliced celery
1/2 cup chopped green bell pepper
1 small onion, chopped
1 clove garlic, minced
1 tablespoon red wine vinegar
3 cups peeled, chopped tomatoes

STEPS

1. Coat a nonstick skillet with cooking spray. Place over medium heat until hot. Add the onion, celery, bell pepper, and garlic. Sauté for 6 minutes. Add the tomatoes, vinegar, and black pepper.

2. Bring to a boil. Cover, reduce the heat, and simmer for 16 minutes, stirring occasionally.

3. Serve!

NUTRITION FACTS

Calories: 29 |Fat: 0 g|Carbohydrates: 7 g|Fiber: 1 g|Protein: 1 g|Sodium: 10 mg|Cholesterol: 0 mg

GRILLED TOMATOES

SERVES FOR
2 PEOPLE

INGREDIENTS

2 large ripe red tomatoes, halved
horizontally
Pinch salt
Pinch freshly ground black pepper

STEPS

1. Place the tomatoes on a grill, put sides facing up. Sprinkle with salt and pepper.

2. Broil for 10 minutes.

3. Serve!

NUTRITION FACTS

Calories: 38 |Fat: 1 g|Carbohydrates: 8 g|Fiber: 2 g|Protein: 2 g|Sodium: 16 mg|Cholesterol: 0 mg

BROILED TOMATO WITH PESTO

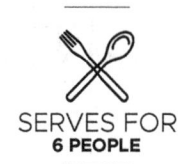

INGREDIENTS

1/4 cup freshly grated Parmesan cheese
1 cup chopped fresh basil leaves
2 cloves garlic
2 tablespoons extra-virgin olive oil
2 tablespoons pine nuts
3 fresh tomatoes

STEPS

1. Cut the tomatoes in half. Combine the olive oil, garlic, basil, Parmesan, and pine nuts in a blender. Puree until smooth. Spoon the mixture onto the top of each tomato half. Place the tomatoes on a broiler pan and broil for about 7 minutes.

2. Serve!

NUTRITION FACTS

Calories: 90 |Fat: 7 g|Carbohydrates: 4 g|Fiber: 1 g|Protein: 3 g|Sodium: 68 mg|Cholesterol: 3 mg

CILANTRO SAUCE

INGREDIENTS

1 tablespoon fresh lime juice
1 teaspoon light soy sauce
1 small clove garlic
3/4 cup reduced-fat mayonnaise
3/4 cup loosely packed cilantro leaves

STEPS

1. Place the mayonnaise, lime juice, cilantro, soy sauce, and garlic in a blender.

2. Blend until smooth.

3. Serve!

NUTRITION FACTS

Calories: 36 |Fat: 3 g|Carbohydrates: 3 g|Fiber: 0 g|Protein: 0 g|Sodium: 104 mg|Cholesterol: 4 mg

LEMON ZEST RICOTTA CRÈME

INGREDIENTS

1/4 teaspoon grated lemon zest
1/4 teaspoon vanilla extract
1/2 cup part-skim ricotta cheese
1 package sugar substitute

STEPS

1. Mix together the ricotta, vanilla extract, lemon zest, and sugar substitute in a dessert bowl.

2. Serve chilled!

NUTRITION FACTS

Calories: 178 |Fat: 10 g|Carbohydrates: 7 g|Fiber: 0 g|Protein: 14 g|Sodium: 155 mg|Cholesterol: 38 mg

ALMOND RICOTTA CRÈME

SERVES FOR
1 PEOPLE

INGREDIENTS

1/4 teaspoon almond extract
1/2 cup part-skim ricotta cheese
1 teaspoon slivered toasted almonds
1 package sugar substitute

STEPS

1. Mix together the almond extract, ricotta, and sugar substitute in a dessert bowl.

2. Serve chilled and garnish with toasted almonds.

NUTRITION FACTS

Calories: 192 |Fat: 11 g|Carbohydrates: 8 g|Fiber: 0 g|Protein: 15 g|Sodium: 155 mg|Cholesterol: 38 mg

VANILLA RICOTTA CRÈME

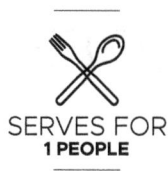

SERVES FOR
1 PEOPLE

INGREDIENTS

1/4 teaspoon vanilla extract
1/2 cup part-skim ricotta cheese
1 package sugar substitute

STEPS

1. Mix together the ricotta, vanilla extract, and sugar substitute in a dessert bowl.

2. Serve chilled.

NUTRITION FACTS

Calories: 178 |Fat: 10 g|Carbohydrates: 7 g|Fiber: 0 g|Protein: 14 g|Sodium: 155 mg|Cholesterol: 38 mg

COFFE RICOTTA CRÈME

INGREDIENTS

1/4 teaspoon vanilla extract
1/2 cup part-skim ricotta cheese
1/2 teaspoon unsweetened cocoa
powder
1 package sugar substitute
5 mini chocolate chips
Dash espresso powder

STEPS

1. Mix together the cocoa powder, vanilla extract, ricotta, and sugar substitute in a dessert bowl.

2. Serve chilled with a dusting of espresso powder and sprinkled with mini chocolate chips.

NUTRITION FACTS

Calories: 261 |Fat: 14 g|Carbohydrates: 17 g|Fiber: 0 g|Protein: 15 g|Sodium: 177 mg|Cholesterol: 42 mg

POACHED SALMON WITH SPINACH SALAD

INGREDIENTS

1/8 teaspoon freshly ground black
pepper
1/4 teaspoon salt
1/2 pound cleaned fresh spinach
1/2 cup chopped yellow onion
1 tablespoon coarsely chopped flat-leaf
parsley
2 tablespoons extra-virgin olive oil
3 fresh tomatoes, peeled, seeded and
cut into 1/2" pieces
Poached salmon

STEPS

1. In a skillet, heat 1 tablespoon of the oil over medium heat. When hot, sauté the spinach for 2 minutes. Add in the salt and pepper and divide the spinach among 4 plates.

2. Heat the remaining tablespoon of oil in the skillet. Sauté the onion and tomatoes over medium heat, about 6 minutes.

3. Arrange the salmon on the spinach and top with the tomatoes and onion.

4. Garnish with parsley.

5. Serve!

NUTRITION FACTS

Calories: 98 |Fat: 7 g|Carbohydrates: 9 g|Fiber: 2 g|Protein: 2 g|Sodium: 162 mg|Cholesterol: 0 mg

MEATLOAF

INGREDIENTS

1/4 tsp dried oregano
1/4 tsp salt
1/4 cup liquid egg substitute
1/2 cup dry red wine
1/2 cup water
1/2 cup shredded zucchini
1/2 tsp dried basil leaves
1 can no-salt-added tomato paste
1 clove garlic, minced
1 lb ground turkey breast
1 cup oatmeal

STEPS

1. Preheat the oven to 375 degrees F. Combine the wine, water, tomato paste, garlic, basil, oregano, and salt in a saucepan. Bring to a boil, and reduce the heat to low. Simmer, uncovered, for 16 minutes. Set aside.

2. Combine the turkey, egg substitute, oatmeal, zucchini, and 1/2 cup of the tomato mixture in a bowl, mix well. Shape into a loaf, and place in an ungreased 8" x 4" loaf pan. Bake for 40 minutes. Discard any drippings. Pour 1/2 cup of the remaining tomato mixture over the top of the loaf. Bake for 13 minutes longer. Remove to a serving platter. Cool for 5 minutes before slicing.

3. Serve the remaining tomato sauce on the side.

NUTRITION FACTS

Calories: 188 |Fat: 3 g|Carbohydrates: 12 g|Fiber: 2 g|Protein: 12 g|Sodium: 244 mg|Cholesterol: 39 mg

LEMON COUSCOUS CHICKEN

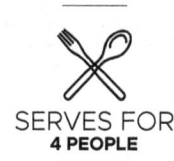

INGREDIENTS

1/4 tsp lemon peel
1 package Near East Roasted Garlic &
Olive Oil Couscous mix
1 Tbsp extra virgin olive oil
1 1/2 cup chopped cooked chicken
1 1/2 cup water
2 cup broccoli florets
2 tbsp juice lemon

STEPS

1. In a skillet, bring to boil the oil, water, broccoli, and contents of the spice sack from the couscous mix. Stir in the couscous, lemon juice, chicken, and lemon peel.

2. Remove from the heat. Cover, and let stand for 5 minutes. Fluff lightly with a fork.

3. Serve cold!

NUTRITION FACTS

Calories: 311 |Fat: 7 g|Carbohydrates: 39 g|Fiber: 3 g|Protein: 24 g|Sodium: 476 mg|Cholesterol: 45 mg

LIME SOUP

INGREDIENTS

1/4 cup lime juice
1/4 cup fresh cilantro, chopped
1/4 teaspoon salt
1/2 cup onion
1/1 teaspoon black pepper
1 medium tomato
1 tablespoon olive oil
1 bay leaf
1-1/2 cups chicken breast, cooked
2 corn tortillas, 6" size
2 Serrano chili peppers
4 cups low-sodium chicken broth
8 cloves garlic
Nonstick cooking spray

STEPS

1. Preheat oven to 425 F.

2. Finely chop onion and cilantro and mince garlic cloves. Thinly slice chili peppers. Cut the tomato in half and remove skin and seeds. Shred chicken.

3. Cut tortillas into thin strips. Arrange the tortilla strips on a baking sheet and spray with cooking spray. Bake for 4 minutes. Remove from oven and place onto a plate to cool.

4. Heat oil in a saucepan over medium heat. Add onion, garlic, and chili peppers. Cook until the onions are translucent.

5. Add tomato, broth, chicken, salt, and bay leaf. Simmer for about 10 minutes.

6. Add lime juice and cilantro. Season with black pepper.

7. Serve with tortilla strips sprinkled on top.

NUTRITION FACTS

Calories: 214 |Fat: 10 g|Carbohydrates: 12 g|Fiber: 1.6 g|Protein: 20 g|Sodium: 246 mg

ROAST BEEF

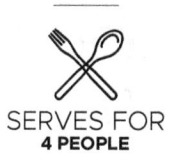

INGREDIENTS

1/2 red onion, sliced
1 1/4 cup reduced-fat cream cheese
4 flour tortillas (9"-10")
4 spinach leaves
8 oz roast beef, sliced

STEPS

1. For each wrap, spread a small amount of the cream cheese over the surface of a tortilla. Layer the spinach, onion, and roast beef. Roll, and fold.

2. Serve!

NUTRITION FACTS

Calories: 300|Fat: 3 g|Carbohydrates: 42 g|Fiber: 3 g|Protein: 13 g|Sodium: 659 mg|Cholesterol: 21 mg

CHOCOLATE DIPPED APRICOTS

INGREDIENTS

1 Tbsp chopped pistachios
2 oz bittersweet chocolate
24 dried apricots

STEPS

1. Put on microwave the chocolate on high for 2 minutes, stirring halfway through, until completely melted. Dip the apricots halfway into the chocolate.

2. Let the excess drip off. Place the apricots onto wax paper. Sprinkle the pistachios over the chocolate-covered portions, and place them in the refrigerator until the chocolate is set.

3. Serve!

NUTRITION FACTS

Calories: 99 |Fat: 3 g|Carbohydrates: 17 g|Fiber: 2 g|Protein: 1 g|Sodium: 1 mg|Cholesterol: 0 mg

SPINACH STUFFED SALMON FILLETS

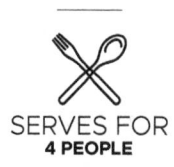

INGREDIENTS

1 tablespoon chopped dry-packed sun-dried tomatoes
1 tablespoon pine nuts
10 ounces baby spinach, coarsely chopped
2 tablespoons prepared pesto
Pinch salt
Pinch freshly ground black pepper
4 salmon fillets

STEPS

1. Heat the oven to 425 degrees F. Make a slit two-thirds of the way through the center of each fillet making sure not to cut all the way through. Season each fillet with salt and pepper. In a bowl, combine the pesto, spinach, tomatoes, and pine nuts. Spoon 1/3 cup of the mixture into each slit.

2. Arrange the fillets on a broiler pan coated with cooking spray. Roast for 10 minutes.

3. Serve!

NUTRITION FACTS

Calories: 329 |Fat: 20 g|Carbohydrates: 4 g|Fiber: 3 g|Protein: 32 g|Sodium: 213 mg|Cholesterol: 86 mg

GRILLED YELLOWFIN TUNA WITH WITHE BEANS

SERVES FOR
4 PEOPLE

INGREDIENTS

1/4 teaspoon crushed garlic
1/4 cup water
1/2 lemon juice
1/2 tablespoon dried oregano
1 teaspoon fresh basil, chopped
1 teaspoon parsley, chopped
2 ounces olive oil
6 ounces sushi-grade yellow fin tuna
12 ounces cooked white beans
Salt
Black pepper

STEPS

1. Sprinkle the tuna with salt and pepper and grill each side for 1 minute. Set aside to cool.

2. Mix the olive oil, water, lemon juice, garlic, basil, oregano, and beans in a cold mixing bowl and let marinate for 2 hours in the refrigerator.

3. To serve, bring the salad to room temperature and place it in the middle of a shallow bowl. Slice the tuna thinly, and lay it on top of the bean mixture.

4. Garnish the plate with the chopped parsley.

5. Serve!

NUTRITION FACTS

Calories: 299 |Fat: 15 g|Carbohydrates: 23 g|Fiber: 10 g|Protein: 18 g|Sodium: 19 mg|Cholesterol: 19 mg

SALMON SOUP

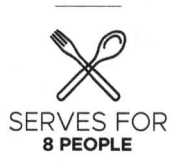

SERVES FOR
8 PEOPLE

INGREDIENTS

1/8 teaspoon black pepper
1/4 cup cornstarch
1/4 cup water
1/2 cup celery
1/2 cup onion
1 medium carrot
1 pound sockeye salmon, cooked
2 tablespoons unsalted butter
2 cups reduced-sodium chicken broth
2 cups 1% low-fat milk

STEPS

1. Chop onion, celery, and carrot.

2. Melt the butter in a 3-quart saucepan on a stovetop burner set to medium heat. Add the vegetables to the saucepan and cook until tender.

3. Add the pre-cooked salmon chunks to the pan.

4. Stir in the milk, chicken broth, and black pepper. Bring mixture to a near-boil, but do not boil. Reduce heat to simmer.

5. Combine the water and cornstarch. Slowly pour into broth mixture, stirring, until the soup is thickened.

6. Simmer for another 6 minutes. Serve warm!

NUTRITION FACTS

Calories: 155 |Fat: 7 g|Carbohydrates: 9 g|Fiber: 0.5 g|Protein: 14 g|Sodium: 113 mg

CHICKEN HONEY NUT STIR FRY

SERVES FOR
6 PEOPLE

INGREDIENTS

1/4 cup cashews
1/4 cup minced green onions
1 tablespoon honey
1 teaspoon minced fresh ginger root
1 tablespoon cornstarch
1 1/2 pounds skinless, boneless chicken breast halves-cut into strips
2 teaspoons peanut oil
2 stalks celery, chopped
2 carrots, peeled and diagonally sliced
3 tablespoons light soy sauce
3/4 cup orange juice

STEPS

1. Heat 1 teaspoon of the oil in a wok over high heat. Add the carrots and celery and stir fry for 2 minutes. Add remaining 1 teaspoon oil, then add the chicken and stir fry for 6 more minutes.

2. In a bowl, dissolve the cornstarch into the orange juice. Mix in the honey, soy sauce, and ginger. Add this sauce to the wok and cook over medium heat until thickened.

3. Garnish with cashews and green onions.

4. Serve!

NUTRITION FACTS

Calories: 235 |Fat: 7.9 g|Carbohydrates: 13 g|Fiber: 1.2 g|Protein: 27 g|Sodium: 536 mg|Cholesterol: 69 mg

SPRING VEGETABLE SOUP

SERVES FOR
5 PEOPLE

INGREDIENTS

1/4 teaspoon salt
1/2 cup frozen corn
1/2 cup onion
1/2 cup carrots
1/2 cup mushrooms
1/2 cup frozen corn
1 cup fresh green beans
1 medium Roma tomato
1 teaspoon dried oregano leaves
1 teaspoon garlic powder
2 tablespoons olive oil
3/4 cup celery
4 cups low-sodium vegetable broth

STEPS

1. Remove tips and strings from the green beans and cut them into 2-inch pieces. Dice the onion, carrots, celery, mushrooms, and tomato.

2. In a pot heat the olive oil and sauté the celery and onion until tender.

3. Add the remaining ingredients and bring to a boil. Reduce heat to a simmer and cook for 65 minutes.

4. Serve!

NUTRITION FACTS

Calories: 114 |Fat: 6 g|Carbohydrates: 13 g|Fiber: 3.4 g|Protein: 2 g|Sodium: 262 mg

GRILLED PORK CHOPS WITH CHIVE CREAM

SERVES FOR
4 PEOPLE

INGREDIENTS

1/2 teaspoon ground white pepper
1 teaspoon salt
1 shallots, crushed
2 tablespoons vegetable oil
4 large pork chops
CHIVE CREAM:
1/8 teaspoon ground white pepper
1/4 teaspoon lemon extract
1/4 teaspoon salt
1/4 cup minced fresh chives
1 cup whipping cream

STEPS

1. In a shallow pan, stir together oil, shallots, salt, and pepper. Place pork chops in the pan, coat with marinade on both sides, and let rest for 30 minutes.

2. Chive Cream: In a saucepan over medium heat, place cream and lemon extract. Simmer until reduced by about one-third; keep warm over low heat. Just before serving, season with salt and pepper, then stir chives into the warm cream sauce.

3. Prepare a charcoal fire or preheat broiler. Place pork chops on the grill, about 4 inches from heat, and cook until browned on one side for about 4 minutes. Turn and cook the second side until lightly browned and slightly firm.

4. Serve chops immediately, and garnish with Chive Cream.

NUTRITION FACTS

Calories: 906 |Fat: 65 g|Carbohydrates: 4 g|Fiber: 0.3 g|Protein: 71 g|Sodium: 897 mg|Cholesterol: 279 mg

APPLE WALNUT CHICKEN SALAD

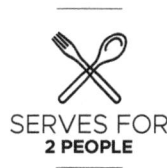

SERVES FOR
2 PEOPLE

INGREDIENTS

1/3 cup prepared low-sugar Italian dressing
1/2 cup chopped celery
1 tablespoon raisins
2 ounces chopped walnuts
3/4 cup chopped apple
5 ounces cooked chicken breast, cut into 1/2" to 3/4" chunks
Bibb Lettuce

STEPS

1. In a bowl, gently stir together the chicken, apple, celery, walnuts, and raisins.

2. Sprinkle dressing over the mixture and toss gently to coat.

3. Serve on a bed of Bibb lettuce.

NUTRITION FACTS

Calories: 444 |Fat: 25 g|Carbohydrates: 33 g|Fiber: 8 g|Protein: 27 g|Sodium: 391 mg|Cholesterol: 63 mg

ORIENTAL CABBAGE SALAD

SERVES FOR
4 PEOPLE

INGREDIENTS

1/2 small head green cabbage
2 tablespoons dark sesame oil
2 tablespoons rice wine vinegar
2 tablespoons sesame seeds, toasted
3 scallions, chopped

STEPS

1. Combine the scallions, cabbage, oil, and vinegar. Toss well and chill until ready to serve.

2. Add the sesame seeds and toss again before serving.

NUTRITION FACTS

Calories: 103 |Fat: 9 g|Carbohydrates: 5 g|Fiber: 2 g|Protein: 2 g|Sodium: 15 mg|Cholesterol: 0 mg

EDAMAME SALAD

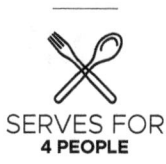

SERVES FOR
4 PEOPLE

INGREDIENTS

1/8 teaspoon fresh ground pepper
1/4 teaspoon salt
1/4 cup seasoned rice vinegar
1 tablespoon vegetable oil
1 bunch radishes cut in half and thinly sliced
1 cup loosely packed chopped fresh cilantro leaves
16 oz. frozen shelled edamame

STEPS

1. Toss the edamame, radishes, vinegar, oil, pepper, salt, and cilantro together in a bowl.

2. If edamame is not readily available, you may substitute it with chickpeas.

3. Serve chilled!

NUTRITION FACTS

Calories: 224 |Fat: 12 g|Carbohydrates: 18 g|Fiber: 6 g|Protein: 15 g|Sodium: 479 mg|Cholesterol: 0 mg

OATMEAL PANCAKE

SERVES FOR
1 PEOPLE

INGREDIENTS

1/4 cup low-fat cottage cheese
1/4 teaspoon cinnamon
1/4 teaspoon nutmeg
1/2 cup old-fashioned oatmeal
1 teaspoon vanilla
4 egg whites

STEPS

1. Process the cottage cheese, oatmeal, vanilla extract, egg whites, cinnamon, and nutmeg in a blender until smooth.

2. Sprinkle a nonstick skillet with cooking spray. Add the batter and cook over medium heat until both sides are lightly browned.

3. You can garnish the pancake with low-sugar syrup!

4. Serve!

NUTRITION FACTS

Calories: 288 |Fat: 4 g|Carbohydrates: 32 g|Fiber: 5 g|Protein: 29 g|Sodium: 451 mg|Cholesterol: 5 mg

SAUCE CHICKEN

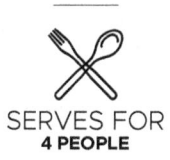

SERVES FOR
4 PEOPLE

INGREDIENTS

1/2 cup fat-free sour cream
1 teaspoon ground cumin
1 pound boneless, skinless chicken
breast, cut into 1" pieces
2 large egg whites
2 tablespoons extra-virgin olive oil
3 Tablespoons chili powder
8 ounces chunky tomato salsa
8 cups finely shredded iceberg lettuce
Cilantro sprigs

STEPS

1. Divide the lettuce among 4 individual plates, cover, and set aside. In a bowl, combine the cumin, and chili powder. Add the chicken, turning to coat. Lift the chicken from the bowl, shaking off the excess coating. Dip the chicken into the egg whites, then coat again with the remaining dry mixture.

2. Heat oil in a wide nonstick frying pan. When the oil is hot, add the chicken and stir-fry gently for 8 minutes.

3. Remove the chicken from the pan and keep warm. Pour the salsa into the pan; reduce the heat to medium and cook, stirring, until the salsa is heated through and slightly thickened.

4. Arrange the chicken over the lettuce; sprinkle with the salsa and sour cream.

5. Garnish with cilantro sprigs.

6. Serve!

NUTRITION FACTS

Calories: 266 |Fat: 10 g|Carbohydrates: 12 g|Fiber: 5 g|Protein: 32 g|Sodium: 457 mg|Cholesterol: 66 mg

BROCCOLI SALAD WITH OLIVES

INGREDIENTS

1/4 teaspoon pepper
1/3 cup olive oil
1/2 teaspoon salt
1 large garlic clove
1 tablespoon capers, drained, rinsed
1 small head broccoli, separated into florets
2 green onions, thinly sliced
2 tablespoons white wine vinegar
3 celery stalks, thinly sliced
6 pimiento-stuffed Spanish olives, sliced

STEPS

1. Cook broccoli in lightly salted boiling water for 6 minutes. Drain and rinse under cold water.

2. In a blender, add garlic, capers, vinegar, salt, and pepper. With the motor running, add oil in a thin, steady stream; blend until smooth. Pour dressing into a large salad bowl.

3. Thinly slice broccoli florets, and add to dressing. Mix in green onions, celery, and olives.

4. Toss gently to coat evenly with dressing.

5. Serve!

NUTRITION FACTS

Calories: 220 |Fat: 18 g|Carbohydrates: 9 g|Fiber: 3.2 g|Protein: 2.7 g

CAULIFLOWER SALAD

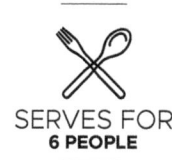

SERVES FOR
6 PEOPLE

INGREDIENTS

1/4 cup mayonnaise
1/2 teaspoon dried mustard
1 very finely chopped jalapeno pepper
1 medium head cauliflower, broken into small florets
2 tablespoons lemon juice
2 packets sugar substitute
3 green onions, chopped
Salt and pepper

STEPS

1. Cook cauliflower in a pot of boiling salted water for 10 minutes. Drain and rinse under cold water; pat dry.

2. In a mixing bowl, mix lemon juice, mayonnaise, sugar substitute, and mustard. Add cauliflower, green onion, and jalapeno pepper. Mix well until vegetables are evenly coated with dressing. Add salt and pepper to taste.

3. Chill 20 minutes in the fridge for flavors to blend.

4. Serve!

NUTRITION FACTS

Calories: 129 |Fat: 11 g|Carbohydrates: 6 g|Fiber: 3.4 g|Protein: 2.5 g

RED CABBAGE

INGREDIENTS

1/4 teaspoon ground black pepper
1/4 cup water
1/4 cup red wine vinegar
1 medium fresh red cabbage, shredded
1 cup fresh onion, chopped
2 tablespoons brown sugar
2 tablespoons unsalted butter
3 cups fresh apples, peeled, cored,
sliced

STEPS

1. Preheat oven to 325 degrees F.

2. Grease a casserole dish.

3. Mix the red cabbage, onion, apples, pepper, water, vinegar, except butter in a bowl. Transfer to the casserole dish. Dot with butter.

4. Cover casserole dish and cook at 325 degrees F for 2 hours.

5. Serve!

NUTRITION FACTS

Calories: 79 |Fat: 3 g|Carbohydrates: 13 g|Fiber: 2 g|Protein: 1 g|Sodium: 13 mg

CHICKEN MARSALA FLORENTINE

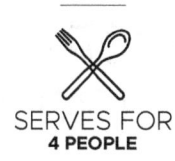

INGREDIENTS

1/4 cup flour
1/2 cup fresh spinach
1 cup marsala wine
1 container sliced portabello mushrooms
1 Tablespoon dried oregano
2 Tablespoons olive oil
3/4 cup butter
3/4 sun dried tomatoes
6 thin sliced chicken breasts

STEPS

1. In a bowl, mix flour and oregano.

2. Coat chicken breasts with flour mixture. In a frying pan, cook chicken with olive oil over medium heat. Cook until done and set aside.

3. In the same frying pan, melt butter and add marsala wine. Once melted, add mushrooms and sun-dried tomatoes. Let simmer for 12 minutes, stirring occasionally.

4. Mix in spinach and add the chicken back to the pan. Cover and allow to cook for an additional 5 minutes.

5. Serve!

NUTRITION FACTS

Calories: 712 |Fat: 48 g|Carbohydrates: 11 g|Fiber: 1 g|Protein: 58 g|Sodium: 777 mg|Cholesterol: 245 mg

CHOP-CHOP
CHICKEN SALAD

INGREDIENTS

Salad:
1/4 cup chopped macadamia nuts
1 cup cucumber, peeled and cut in 1/4"
dice
1 cup zucchini, in 1/4" dice
1 cup red peppers, in 1/4" dice
1 cup celery, in 1/4" dice
2 medium heads endive, sliced
lengthwise in narrow strips
2 tablespoons fresh cilantro, chopped
4 boneless, skinless chicken breast
halves, grilled and cut into
6 cups chopped Napa cabbage

Dressing:
1/4 cup low-sodium soy sauce
1/4 cup fresh lemon juice
1 tablespoon toasted sesame oil
1 packet sugar substitute

STEPS

1. For the dressing, in a bowl whisk lemon juice, soy sauce, sesame oil, and sugar substitute until well combined; set aside.

2. In a bowl, mix chicken, vegetables, and cilantro. Pour in dressing; mix well. Let the salad sit for 10 minutes for flavors to blend. Divide evenly into 4 plates.

3. Garnish with macadamia nuts.

4. Serve!

NUTRITION FACTS

Calories: 320 |Fat: 13 g|Carbohydrates: 11 g|Fiber: 1.5 g|Protein: 38 g

QUICK CREAMY COLESLAW

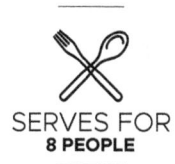

INGREDIENTS

1/2 cup sour cream
1 teaspoon celery seed
1 teaspoon salt
1 medium cabbage, halved and cored
2 carrots
2 tablespoons cider vinegar
2 packets sugar substitute
3/4 cup mayonnaise

STEPS

1. Cut cabbage halves in half and thinly slice. Transfer to a bowl. Coarsely grate carrots and put on the cabbage and mix well.

2. In another bowl, whisk together sour cream, mayonnaise, celery, cider vinegar, sugar substitute, and salt. Pour dressing over vegetables. Mix until thoroughly combined.

3. Refrigerate at least 20 minutes before serving for flavors to blend. Serve!

NUTRITION FACTS

Calories: 143 |Fat: 19 g|Carbohydrates: 8 g|Fiber: 2.5 g|Protein: 2.1 g

LEMON CHICKEN

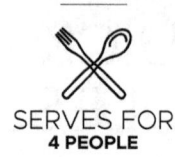

INGREDIENTS

1/4 cup chicken broth, low sodium
1/4 cup water
1/4 teaspoon ground black pepper
1 teaspoon fresh basil, chopped
1 teaspoon dried oregano
1 pound chicken breast, boneless, skinless
1 tablespoon lemon juice
2 cloves garlic, minced
2 tablespoons butter, unsalted

STEPS

1. Combine oregano and ground black pepper in a bowl. Rub the mixture on the chicken.

2. Melt the butter in a skillet over medium heat. Brown the chicken in the melted butter and then transfer the chicken to the slow cooker.

3. Place water, chicken broth, lemon juice, and garlic in the skillet. Bring it to a boil so it loosens the browned bits from the skillet. Pour over the chicken.

4. Cover, set slow cooker on high for 2 hours.

5. Add basil and baste the chicken. Cover, cook on high for an additional 25 minutes.

6. Serve!

NUTRITION FACTS

Calories: 197 |Fat: 9 g|Carbohydrates: 1 g|Fiber: 3 g|Protein: 26 g|Sodium: 57 mg

CRUNCHY GREEN BEAN

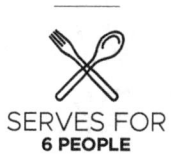

SERVES FOR
6 PEOPLE

INGREDIENTS

1/4 cup gorgonzola, crumbled
1/2 cup plain unsalted tortilla chips, crushed
1/2 cup panko breadcrumbs
2 tablespoons hot sauce
2 tablespoons butter, unsalted, melted
2 tablespoons green onions, chopped
12 oz of Fresh String green beans

STEPS

1. Preheat oven to 350 degrees F.

2. Chop green beans to ~2" pieces, steam for 6 minutes in a microwave-safe plate, damp moist paper towel.

3. Mix cut string green beans with the hot sauce. Pour mixture into a casserole dish.

4. Mix gorgonzola, tortilla chips, bread crumbs, butter, and green onions, in a bowl. Sprinkle mixture evenly over string green beans and bake green bean casserole uncovered in the oven for 20 minutes.

5. Serve!

NUTRITION FACTS

Calories: 122 |Fat: 6 g|Carbohydrates: 11 g|Fiber: 2.4 g|Protein: 4 g|Sodium: 221 mg

HAWAIIAN-STYLE PULLED PORK

INGREDIENTS

1/4 teaspoon of sugar
1/3 cup white vinegar
1/2 teaspoon garlic powder
1/2 teaspoon paprika
1/2 teaspoon ground black pepper
1 teaspoon onion powder
1 red onion
2 tablespoons liquid smoke
4 pounds pork roast

STEPS

1. Combine paprika, black pepper, onion, and garlic powder in a bowl.

2. Rub the seasoning blend on all sides of the pork. Place pork into a slow cooker. Sprinkle with liquid smoke.

3. Add enough water to the slow cooker. Cook on high for 4 hours.

4. Remove pork from cooking liquid and shred meat using two forks.

5. Garnish with a mixture of sugar, chopped red onion, and vinegar!

6. Serve!

NUTRITION FACTS

Calories: 285 |Fat: 21 g|Carbohydrates: 1 g|Fiber: 0 g|Protein: 20 g|Sodium: 54 mg

HERB-CRUSTED ROAST LEG OF LAMB

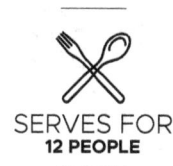

INGREDIENTS

1/2 teaspoon ground black pepper
1/2 cup dry vermouth 1 4-pound leg of lamb
1 cup onions, sliced
1 tablespoon curry powder
3 tablespoons lemon juice
2 cloves garlic, minced

STEPS

1. Preheat oven to 425 degrees F.

2. Place the leg of lamb on a roasting pan. Sprinkle with 1 teaspoon of lemon juice.

3. Make the paste with 2 teaspoons of lemon juice and the rest of the spices. Rub the paste onto the lamb.

4. Roast lamb in 425 degrees F oven for 30 minutes.

5. Drain off fat and add vermouth and onions.

6. Reduce heat to 325 F and cook for an additional 2 hours. Baste leg of lamb frequently. When the internal temperature is 145 F, remove it from the oven and let rest 5 minutes before serving.

NUTRITION FACTS

Calories: 292 |Fat: 20 g|Carbohydrates: 2 g|Fiber: 0 g|Protein: 24 g|Sodium: 157 mg

HERB-CRUSTED PORK LOIN

SERVES FOR
14 PEOPLE

INGREDIENTS

1 boneless pork loin roast
2 tablespoons soy sauce, low sodium
2 tablespoons anise seed
2 tablespoons fennel seed
2 tablespoons caraway seed
2 tablespoons dill seed

STEPS

1. Rub soy sauce over the roast until it's coated all over.

2. In a baking pan, stir together the fennel, anise seed, caraway, and dill seed. Roll pork roast in seeds to coat evenly. Wrap the meat in foil; refrigerate for at least overnight.

3. Preheat the oven to 350 degrees F and remove foil. Place meat fat side up on the rack in an open shallow roasting pan. Insert meat thermometer so the tip is in the center of the thickest part.

4. Roast pork loin in a baking pan for about 35 minutes. A meat thermometer should register 145 F when the roast is done. Let rest 5 minutes. Slice to serve.

NUTRITION FACTS

Calories: 224 |Fat: 13 g|Carbohydrates: 2 g|Fiber: 1.0 g|Protein: 24 g|Sodium: 134 mg

DELICIOUS HOT CRAB DIP

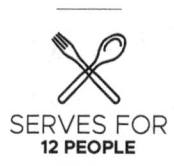

SERVES FOR
12 PEOPLE

INGREDIENTS

1/4 teaspoon pepper
1/4 cup sour cream
1/4 cup mayonnaise
1/2 teaspoon salt
1/2 teaspoon paprika
1 cup cheddar cheese grated
1 teaspoon garlic powder
1 Tablespoon Worcestershire Sauce
1 Tablespoon lemon juice
1 pound lump crab meat canned
8 ounce cream cheese softened

STEPS

1. Preheat your oven to 375 degrees F. In a mixing bowl, combine cream cheese, mayonnaise, sour cream, cheddar cheese, paprika, garlic powder, lemon juice, Worcestershire sauce, salt, and pepper. Stir together until combined and fold in lump crab meat.

2. Spread in a casserole dish and bake for 20 minutes.

3. Serve with tortilla chips!

NUTRITION FACTS

Calories: 178 |Fat: 7 g|Carbohydrates: 2 g|Fiber: 1 g|Protein: 11 g|Sodium: 580 mg|Cholesterol: 51 mg

SPINACH AND ARTICHOKE SALAD

SERVES FOR
4 PEOPLE

INGREDIENTS

1 tablespoon olive oil
1 package spinach - rinsed, stemmed, and dried
1 red onion, thinly sliced
1 jar marinated artichoke hearts
1 cup crumbled feta cheese

STEPS

1. Preheat oven to 300 degrees F.

2. Sprinkle with olive oil on a rimmed baking sheet. Spread spinach leaves in a thick layer covering the baking sheet. Arrange artichokes and onions over the spinach, and drizzle the marinade from the jar over the entire salad. Sprinkle with the cheese.

3. Bake for about 12 minutes.

4. Serve!

NUTRITION FACTS

Calories: 243 |Fat: 20 g|Carbohydrates: 10 g|Fiber: 2 g|Protein: 7.6 g|Sodium: 667 mg|Cholesterol: 33 mg

LEMON PEPPER CHICKEN

INGREDIENTS

1/3 cup all purpose flour
1 tablespoon chopped parsley
1 tablespoon lemon pepper seasoning
2 tablespoons olive oil
2 tablespoons butter
2 teaspoons lemon juice
4 thin cut boneless skinless chicken breasts
Salt to taste

STEPS

1. Mix together the flour, lemon pepper seasoning, and salt to taste. Pour the flour mixture onto a plate.

2. Heat the olive oil in a pan over medium heat.

3. Dredge the chicken breasts in the flour mixture, turning to coat evenly.

4. Place the chicken in the pan and cook for 7 minutes per side.

5. Remove the chicken from the pan and place it on a plate. Cover to keep warm.

6. Melt the butter in the pan, and whisk in the lemon juice. Season with salt to taste.

7. Spoon the sauce over the chicken. Garnish with parsley and serve!

NUTRITION FACTS

Calories: 345 |Fat: 17 g|Carbohydrates: 11 g|Fiber: 1 g|Protein: 36 g|Sodium: 1000mg|Cholesterol: 111 mg

MASHED CARROTS & GINGER

SERVES FOR
3 PEOPLE

INGREDIENTS

1/2 teaspoon fresh ginger, chopped
1/2 teaspoon honey
1/2 teaspoon black pepper
1/2 teaspoon vanilla extract
2 cups baby carrots

STEPS

1. Boil carrots on high heat until carrots are very tender. Lower heat to low and mash carrots with a potato masher.

2. Add the honey, ginger, pepper, and vanilla extract and stir until well-mixed.

3. Serve!

NUTRITION FACTS

Calories: 30 |Fat: 0 g|Carbohydrates: 7 g|Fiber: 2 g|Protein: 1 g|Sodium: 55 mg

PARMESAN AND BASIL CHICKEN SALAD

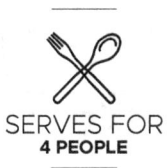

SERVES FOR
4 PEOPLE

INGREDIENTS

1 cup mayonnaise
1 cup chopped fresh basil
2 whole skinless, boneless chicken breasts
2 cloves crushed garlic
2/3 cup grated Parmesan cheese
3 stalks celery, chopped
Salt and pepper to taste

STEPS

1. Season chicken with salt and pepper.

   Roast at 350 degrees F for 45 minutes.

   Let cool, and chop into chunks.

2. In a food processor, puree the garlic, mayonnaise, basil, and celery.

3. Combine the chunked chicken, pureed mixture, and Parmesan cheese; mix.

4. Refrigerate for 15 minutes and serve.

NUTRITION FACTS

Calories: 422 |Fat: 49 g|Carbohydrates: 3.9 g|Fiber: 0.6 g|Protein: 33 g|Sodium: 617 mg|Cholesterol: 100 mg

ROASTED EGGPLANT PURÉE

INGREDIENTS

1/4 cup olive oil
1/2 teaspoon salt
1 1-pound eggplant
2 garlic cloves, pushed through a press
Freshly ground black pepper to taste
Chopped fresh parsley to taste

STEPS

1. Heat oven to 450 degrees F. Cut eggplant on all sides with deep slashes and place on a baking sheet. Roast until soft, about 35 minutes. Set aside until cool enough to handle.

2. Peel eggplant and coarsely chop. Place in a bowl. Mix in oil, garlic, salt, pepper.

3. Garnish with parsley.

4. Serve!

NUTRITION FACTS

Calories: 76 |Fat: 7 g|Carbohydrates: 3.5 g|Fiber: 11.4 g|Protein: 0.6 g

BAKED ROSEMARY CHICKEN

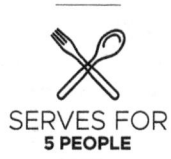

INGREDIENTS

1/2 teaspoon coarse ground black
pepper
1 tablespoon fresh rosemary , chopped
1 teaspoon salt
2 tablespoon lemon juice
2 tablespoons vegetable oil
3 cloves garlic , chopped
5 chicken thighs , bone in and skin on

STEPS

1. Preheat the oven to 400 degrees F.

2. Mix the oil, lemon juice, rosemary,
    garlic, salt, and pepper, place chicken,
    skin side up in a baking pan.

3. Roast for 30 minutes.

4. Serve!

NUTRITION FACTS

Calories: 186 |Fat: 10 g|Carbohydrates: 1 g|Fiber: 1 g|Protein: 22 g|Sodium: 566 mg|Cholesterol: 107 mg

ROSEMARY CHICKEN AND WHITE BEANS

SERVES FOR
4 PEOPLE

INGREDIENTS

1/4 small red onion, thinly sliced
1 15.5-ounce can cannellini beans, rinsed
2 teaspoons Dijon mustard
2 tablespoons red wine vinegar
2 tablespoons chopped fresh rosemary
2 cloves garlic, chopped
4 6-ounce boneless, skinless chicken breasts
4 cups baby arugula
5 tablespoons olive oil
Salt and black pepper

STEPS

1. In a baking dish, whisk the 2 tablespoons of the oil, rosemary, vinegar, garlic, 1/2 teaspoon salt, and 1/4 teaspoon pepper. Add the chicken and turn to coat. Refrigerate, covered, for 20 minutes.

2. Meanwhile, in a bowl, whisk the 2 tablespoons of the remaining oil, mustard, and 1/2 teaspoon each salt and pepper. Add the beans, onion, and arugula, and toss to combine.

3. Heat the remaining tablespoon of oil in a skillet over medium heat. Remove the chicken from the marinade and cook until cooked through, 8 minutes per side.

4. Serve the chicken with the arugula and beans.

NUTRITION FACTS

Calories: 394|Fat: 21 g|Carbohydrates: 11 g|Fiber: 3 g|Protein: 38 g|Sodium: 594 mg|Cholesterol: 94 mg

SALMON-STUFFED ZUCCHINI

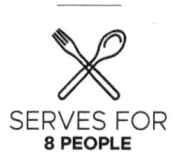

INGREDIENTS

1/4 cup roasted red sweet pepper,
drained and chopped
1/4 cup light mayonnaise
1/3 cup finely chopped green onions
1/2 cup panko bread crumbs
1/2 cup finely shredded Parmesan
cheese
2 tablespoons snipped fresh parsley
1 teaspoon dried Italian seasoning,
crushed
3 2.5 ounces plain skinless, boneless
pink salmon
4 medium zucchini
Lemon wedges

STEPS

1. Preheat broiler. Cut each zucchini in half lengthwise, trim ends. Using a small spoon, scoop out and discard the pulp, leaving 1/4-inch-thick shells. Place zucchini shells, cut sides up, in a shallow baking pan. Broil 4 inches from the heat for 5 minutes.

2. Meanwhile, in a bowl stir the red sweet pepper, green onions, parsley, mayonnaise, and Italian seasoning. Add salmon and bread crumbs. Stir gently to combine.

3. Spoon salmon mixture into broiled zucchini halves. Sprinkle with cheese. Broil for about 4 minutes.

4. Serve with lemon wedges.

NUTRITION FACTS

Calories: 228 |Fat: 11 g|Carbohydrates: 15 g|Fiber: 3 g|Protein: 19 g|Sodium: 558 mg|Cholesterol: 40 mg

SWEET POTATO HASH BROWNS

INGREDIENTS

1/4 cup finely chopped shallot
1/2 teaspoon salt
1/2 teaspoon ground pepper
1 medium clove garlic, grated
3 tablespoons extra-virgin olive oil, divided
5 cups peeled and shredded sweet potato

STEPS

1. Combine the shallot, garlic, sweet potato,1 tablespoon oil, salt, and pepper in a bowl.

2. Heat 1 tablespoon oil in a cast-iron skillet over medium heat. Form three 1/2-cup sweet potato patties in the pan, flattening them with a spatula. Cook the patties, turning once and lowering the heat to low if the pan gets too hot until nicely browned on both sides, for 8 minutes total. Transfer to a baking sheet and cover to keep warm. Repeat with the remaining 1 tablespoon oil and the remaining sweet potato mixture.

3. Serve!

NUTRITION FACTS

Calories: 103 |Fat: 7 g|Carbohydrates: 9 g|Fiber: 1.4 g|Protein: 1 g|Sodium: 208 mg

SCALLOPS WITH PESTO CREAM SAUCE

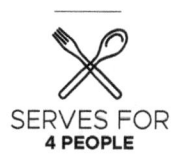

SERVES FOR
4 PEOPLE

INGREDIENTS

1 pound scallops
1 tablespoon pesto
1 tablespoon capers
1 cup heavy whipping cream
2 tablespoons all-purpose flour
2 tablespoons butter
Salt and freshly ground black pepper to taste

STEPS

1. Season the scallops with salt and pepper, then dredge in flour.

2. Melt butter in a skillet over medium heat and add scallops. Cook for 2 minutes for the side. Add pesto and capers; mix well. Stir in heavy cream and bring to a boil.

3. Remove from heat and serve.

NUTRITION FACTS

Calories: 389 |Fat: 30 g|Carbohydrates: 5 g|Fiber: 0.3 g|Protein: 23 g|Sodium: 403 mg|Cholesterol: 144 mg

SIRLOIN TIPS AND MUSHROOMS

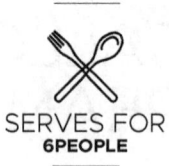

SERVES FOR
6PEOPLE

INGREDIENTS

1 1/2 pounds beef sirloin
3 tablespoons olive oil
3 cloves garlic, minced
3/4 cup red wine
8 ounce tomato sauce
16 ounce mushrooms, with liquid
Salt to taste
Freshly ground pepper

STEPS

1. Cut beef into cubes. In a skillet over medium heat, heat the olive oil and brown beef cubes with the garlic.

2. Add the tomato sauce, the mushrooms with liquid, salt, pepper, and red wine. Cook for 40 minutes.

3. Serve!

NUTRITION FACTS

Calories: 257 |Fat: 13 g|Carbohydrates: 7 g|Fiber: 2 g|Protein: 21 g|Sodium: 555 mg|Cholesterol: 49 mg

SOUTHWESTERN CHICKEN

SERVES FOR
4 PEOPLE

INGREDIENTS

1/2 teaspoon salt
1/2 teaspoon paprika
1 teaspoon chili powder
2 teaspoons garlic powder
2 teaspoons lime juice
4 boneless skinless chicken breast
halves (4 ounces each)

STEPS

1. In a bowl, combine the chili powder, garlic powder, salt, and paprika. Rub over both sides of the chicken.

2. In a skillet coated with cooking spray, brown chicken on both sides; sprinkle with the lime juice. Cover and cook for 8 minutes.

3. Serve!

NUTRITION FACTS

Calories: 130 |Fat: 3 g|Carbohydrates: 2 g|Fiber: 0 g|Protein: 23 g|Sodium: 357 mg|Cholesterol: 63 mg

CHICKPEAS WITH SPINACH

INGREDIENTS

1/2 bag baby leaf spinach
1 rasher lean back bacon
1 thinly sliced garlic clove
1 tbsp wine vinegar
3 tbsp canned chickpeas, drained and
washed
Salt and black pepper

STEPS

1. Cut the bacon rasher into strips and
    cook in a hot non-stick pan with the
    garlic clove. Add the wine vinegar,
    chickpeas, and spinach, stirring until
    wilted.

2. Season with salt and pepper.

3. Serve!

NUTRITION FACTS

Calories: 97 |Fat: 3 g|Carbohydrates: 9 g|Fiber: 2 g|Protein: 9 g|Sugars: 0 g|Sodium: 1.54 g

SPINACH STUFFED CHICKEN BREASTS

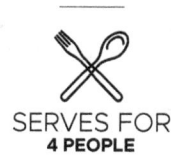

INGREDIENTS

1/4 teaspoon garlic powder
1/4 teaspoon onion powder
1/4 cup grated Parmesan
1/2 teaspoon red pepper flakes
1 teaspoon garlic, minced
1 tablespoon olive oil
1 tesapoon paprika
1 teaspoon salt, divided
1 1/2cups chopped fresh spinach
2 tablespoons mayonnaise
4 chicken breasts
4 ounces cream cheese, softened

STEPS

1. Preheat oven to 400 degrees F.

2. Place the chicken breasts on a cutting board and sprinkle with olive oil.

3. Add the paprika, 1/2 teaspoon salt, onion powder, and garlic powder, to a bowl and stir to combine. Sprinkle evenly over both sides of the chicken.

4. Use a sharp knife to cut a pocket into the side of each chicken breast. Set chicken aside.

5. Add the spinach, Parmesan, cream cheese, mayonnaise, garlic, red pepper, and remaining 1/2 teaspoon of salt to a mixing bowl and stir well to combine.

6. Spoon the spinach mixture into each chicken breast evenly.

7. Place the chicken breasts in a baking dish. Bake, uncovered, for 20 minutes or until chicken is golden.

8. Serve!

NUTRITION FACTS

Calories: 407 |Fat: 24 g|Carbohydrates: 3 g|Fiber: 1 g|Protein: 41 g|Sodium: 873 mg|Cholesterol: 139 mg

JAPANESE-STYLE SESAME GREEN BEANS

SERVES FOR
4 PEOPLE

INGREDIENTS

1 tablespoon canola oil
1 pound fresh green beans, washed
1 tablespoon soy sauce
1 tablespoon toasted sesame seeds
1 1/2 teaspoons sesame oil

STEPS

1. Warm a skillet wok over medium heat. When the skillet is hot, pour in canola and sesame oils, then place whole green beans into the skillet. Stir the beans to coat with oil.

2. Cook for about 12 minutes. Remove from heat, and stir in soy sauce; cover, and let sit for about 3 minutes. Transfer to a serving platter, and garnish with toasted sesame seeds.

3. Serve!

NUTRITION FACTS

Calories: 97 |Fat: 6.6 g|Carbohydrates: 9 g|Fiber: 4 g|Protein: 2.7 g|Sodium: 232 mg

STUFFED CELERY

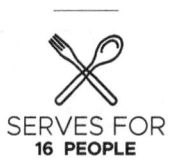

INGREDIENTS

1/4 cup chopped walnuts
1 bunch celery, cut into bite-size pieces
2 tablespoons sour cream
8 ounce cream cheese, softened
20 green olives with pimento, chopped

STEPS

1. In a bowl, mix the sour cream, and cream cheese. Stir in the walnuts and chopped olives. Spread filling onto the celery pieces.

2. Serve!

NUTRITION FACTS

Calories: 76 |Fat: 7 g|Carbohydrates: 1.8 g|Fiber: 0.6 g|Protein: 1.7 g|Sodium: 186 mg|Cholesterol: 16 mg

STUFFED
MEATBALLS

INGREDIENTS

1/2 tsp pepper
1/2 cup almond flour
1 lb ground beef
1 lb sausage
1 egg
1 tbsp dried minced onion
1 tsp Italian seasoning
1 tsp garlic powder
1 tsp salt
16 oz mozzarella cheese cut into 24 cubes

STEPS

1. Preheat oven to 400 degrees F. Spray a sheet pan with cooking spray

2. Combine the almond flour, beef, sausage, egg onion, garlic, Italiana seasoning, salt, and pepper in a bowl and mix thoroughly. Make 24 meatballs. Insert one cube of mozzarella into each meatball and enclose it in the meat. Put the mozzarella stuffed meatballs on the prepared pan.

3. Bake for 30 minutes.

4. Serve!

NUTRITION FACTS

Calories: 405|Fat: 33 g|Carbohydrates: 4 g|Fiber: 1 g|Protein: 37 g|Sodium: 1044 mg|Cholesterol: 137 mg

TOMATO MOZZARELLA SALAD

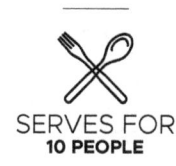

SERVES FOR
10 PEOPLE

INGREDIENTS

1/8 teaspoon ground black pepper
1/4 cup olive oil
1/4 cup balsamic vinegar
1/4 teaspoon salt
1/4 cup minced fresh basil
3 large tomatoes, sliced
8 ounces mozzarella cheese, sliced

STEPS

1. Place tomato slices, alternating with mozzarella slices, on a large serving platter.

2. Combine the oil, balsamic vinegar, salt, and pepper in a jar with a fitting lid; shake well.

3. Sprinkle the tomatoes and mozzarella with the blend.

4. Garnish with basil. Serve!

NUTRITION FACTS

Calories: 199 |Fat: 15 g|Carbohydrates: 6 g|Fiber: 1.1 g|Protein: 10 g|Sodium: 338 mg|Cholesterol: 24 mg

TRI-COLOR SALAD

INGREDIENTS

Dressing:
1/4 teaspoon pepper
1/2 teaspoon lemon juice
1/2 teaspoon salt
1 tablespoon balsamic vinegar
3 tablespoons olive oil
Salad:
1/2 small head radicchio, cut into bite-sized pieces
1/2 small head Bibb lettuce, cut into bite-sized pieces
1 head endive, thinly sliced on the diagonal

STEPS

1. In a salad bowl, mix the olive oil, lemon juice, balsamic vinegar, salt, and pepper.

2. Add the radicchio, the lettuce, and the endive. Toss to coat with dressing.

3. Serve!

NUTRITION FACTS

Calories: 106 |Fat: 10 g|Carbohydrates: 2.5 g|Fiber: 1 g|Protein: 1 g

TURKEY MARSALA

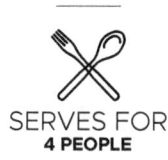

SERVES FOR
4 PEOPLE

INGREDIENTS

1/4 cup all-purpose flour
1/2 teaspoon salt, divided
1/2 teaspoon pepper, divided
1/2 pound sliced fresh mushrooms
1/2 cup reduced-sodium chicken broth
1/2 cup Marsala wine
1 tablespoon olive oil
1 tablespoon butter
1 teaspoon lemon juice
20 ounces turkey breast tenderloins

STEPS

1. Mix flour, 1/4 teaspoon salt, and 1/4 teaspoon pepper. Cut each tenderloin crosswise in half; pound each piece with a meat mallet to 3/4-in. thickness. Toss with flour mixture; shake off excess.

2. In a nonstick skillet, heat oil over medium heat. Add turkey; cook for about 8 minutes per side. Remove from pan; keep warm.

3. In the same skillet, heat butter over medium heat; saute mushrooms, for 5 minutes. Stir in broth and wine. Bring to a boil, stirring to loosen browned bits from pan; cook until liquid is reduced by half, for about 13 minutes.

4. Stir in lemon juice and the remaining salt and pepper.

5. Serve with turkey!

NUTRITION FACTS

Calories: 295 |Fat: 8 g|Carbohydrates: 12 g|Fiber: 1 g|Protein: 36 g|Sodium: 482 mg

GRILLED SALMON RADICCHIO WRAPS

INGREDIENTS

Pico de Gallo:
1/2 red bell pepper, seeded and diced
1/2 red onion, chopped
1 tomato, seeded and diced
1 lime, juiced
Cream Sauce:
1/2 teaspoon seasoning blend
2 tablespoons skim milk
2/3 cup plain Greek yogurt
Wraps:
1 pound skinless grilled salmon, cut into chunks
12 leaves whole radicchio leaves

STEPS

1. Combine the red bell pepper, onion, tomato, and lime juice in a bowl to make pico de gallo.

2. Whisk skim milk, Greek yogurt, and seasoning blend together in another bowl to make the cream sauce.

3. Place some grilled salmon chunks in a radicchio leaf. Top with some pico de gallo and cream sauce. Repeat with remaining salmon and radicchio leaves.

4. Serve!

NUTRITION FACTS

Calories: 306 |Fat: 17 g|Carbohydrates: 7 g|Fiber: 1.3 g|Protein: 28 g|Sodium: 103 mg|Cholesterol: 79 mg

SICILIAN ROASTED CHICKEN

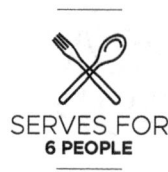

SERVES FOR
6 PEOPLE

INGREDIENTS

1 whole chicken, cut into 8 pieces
1 teaspoon salt
1 teaspoon ground black pepper
1 teaspoon ground paprika
1 teaspoon garlic powder
1 teaspoon dried oregano
Cooking spray

STEPS

1. Preheat oven to 400 degrees F. Grease a pan with cooking spray.

2. Arrange chicken pieces in the baking pan. Sprinkle with paprika, garlic powder, salt, pepper, and oregano over both sides.

3. Roast in the preheated oven until chicken is browned, for about 1 hour and 10 minutes.

4. Serve!

NUTRITION FACTS

Calories:431 |Fat: 25 g|Carbohydrates: 0.9 g|Fiber: 0.4 g|Protein: 46 g|Sodium: 528 mg|Cholesterol: 145 mg

CREAM OF MUSHROOM SOUP

SERVES FOR
6 PEOPLE

INGREDIENTS

1/4 teaspoon dried thyme
1/4 cup butter
1/2 cup finely chopped onion
1/2 teaspoon salt
1/2 teaspoon ground black pepper
1 clove garlic, minced
2 tablespoons sherry
2 cups heavy whipping cream
4 ounce cream cheese
5 cups coarsely chopped fresh mushrooms
32 ounce chicken broth

STEPS

1. Melt butter in a heavy saucepan over medium heat. Add onion, garlic, and mushrooms; cook and stir for 12 minutes. Add salt, pepper, and thyme; cook and stir until combined, about 1 minute. Add and stir in chicken broth, heavy cream, and cream cheese.

2. Reduce heat to a low simmer and pour in sherry. Cook, for about 40 minutes.

3. Serve!

NUTRITION FACTS

Calories: 433 |Fat: 44 g|Carbohydrates: 7.8 g|Fiber: 0.9 g|Protein: 5.9 g|Sodium: 1082mg|Cholesterol: 153 mg

CHICKEN-VEGETABLE SOUP

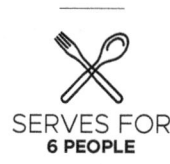

SERVES FOR
6 PEOPLE

INGREDIENTS

6 cups water
2 cups chicken stock
4 medium celery stalks, sliced
3 medium carrots, sliced
1/2 cup chopped yellow onion
2 cloves garlic, minced
2 tablespoons chopped fresh parsley
1 teaspoon ground thyme
1/2 teaspoon paprika
salt and ground black pepper to taste
1 bay leaf
1 pound chopped cooked chicken
4 cups sliced yellow squash

STEPS

1. Combine celery, carrots, onion, garlic, water, stock, parsley, thyme, paprika, salt, black pepper, and bay leaf in a pot. Bring to a simmer, cover, and cook for 30 minutes.

2. Add cooked chicken and squash to the pot and simmer for about 10 minutes more.

3. Serve!

NUTRITION FACTS

Calories: 185 |Fat: 6 g|Carbohydrates: 9 g|Fiber: 3.3 g|Protein: 22 g|Sodium: 350 mg|Cholesterol: 57 mg

BROCCOLI SOUP

SERVES FOR
8 PEOPLE

INGREDIENTS

1/8 teaspoon ground black pepper
1/4 teaspoon salt
1/4 cup freshly squeezed lemon juice
1/4 cup shredded Cheddar cheese
1 tablespoon extra-virgin olive oil
1 large onion, finely chopped
2 cloves garlic, minced
2 pounds broccoli, chopped
5 cups vegetable broth

STEPS

1. Heat oil in a pot over medium heat; once the oil is hot, reduce heat to low. Cook and stir onion and garlic in hot oil for 4 minutes. Add broccoli, season with salt and pepper, and stir. Pour vegetable broth and lemon juice into the pot.

2. Loosely cover the pot and simmer the mixture until the broccoli is tender about 25 minutes. Puree with an immersion blender until smooth.

3. Garnish with Cheddar cheese to serve.

NUTRITION FACTS

Calories: 97 |Fat: 3.6 g|Carbohydrates: 13 g|Fiber: 3.9 g|Protein: 5 g|Sodium: 420 mg|Cholesterol: 4 mg

CAULIFLOWER LEEK SOUP

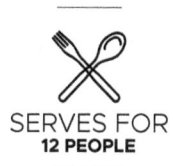

INGREDIENTS

1 cup heavy cream
1 large head cauliflower, chopped
2 tablespoons olive oil
3 tablespoons butter
3 leeks, cut into 1 inch pieces
3 cloves garlic, finely chopped
8 cups vegetable broth
salt and freshly ground black pepper to taste

STEPS

1. Heat the olive oil and butter in a pot over medium heat, and saute the leeks, cauliflower, and garlic for about 10 minutes. Stir in the vegetable broth, and bring the mixture to a boil. Reduce heat, cover, and simmer for 50 minutes.

2. Remove the soup from heat. Blend the soup with an immersion blender. Season with salt and pepper. Mix in the heavy cream, and continue blending until smooth.

3. Serve!

NUTRITION FACTS

Calories: 156 |Fat: 13 g|Carbohydrates: 8 g|Fiber: 2.2 g|Protein: 2.4 g|Sodium: 346 mg|Cholesterol: 34 mg

PUMPKIN SOUP

INGREDIENTS

1 cup heavy cream
1 teaspoon salt
1 tablespoon olive oil
1 small onion, diced
1 1/2 teaspoons pumpkin pie spice
2 cloves garlic, minced
2 tablespoons heavy cream
2 tablespoons zero-calorie brown sugar substitute
2 1/2 cups chicken stock
3 tablespoons crushed walnuts
15 ounce pumpkin puree

STEPS

1. Heat oil in a saucepan over medium heat. Add onion and saute for 3 minutes. Reduce heat to medium-low and add garlic. Saute until the onion is beginning to soften, for 3 more minutes. Stir in sugar substitute, pumpkin pie spice, and salt. Pour in chicken stock and stir to combine. Whisk in pumpkin puree, cover, and simmer over medium-low heat for 12 minutes.

2. Blend soup carefully until smooth using an immersion blender. Stir in 1 cup heavy cream and adjust salt.

3. Garnish with a drizzle of heavy cream and crushed walnuts.

4. Serve!

NUTRITION FACTS

Calories: 244 |Fat: 20 g|Carbohydrates: 9 g|Fiber: 2.6 g|Protein: 7 g|Sodium: 862 mg|Cholesterol: 58 mg

LIME AMBROSIA
FRUIT CUP

SERVES FOR
12 PORTIONS

INGREDIENTS

1/3 cup toasted coconut
1/2 teaspoon ground ginger
1 tablespoon honey
3 teaspoons finely shredded lime peel
3 tablespoons lime juice
8 cups cut up fresh melon, strawberries,
seedless grapes, and peaches

STEPS

1. Place fruit in a large bowl. Combine
   lime juice, lime peel, honey, and ginger
   in a small bowl; pour over the fruit and
   toss.

2. Just before serving, garnish with
   toasted coconut.

NUTRITION FACTS

Calories: 65 |Fat: 1.3 g|Carbohydrates: 13 g|Fiber: 1.6 g|Protein: 1 g|Sodium: 20 mg

QUARK & CUCUMBER TOAST

INGREDIENTS

1 slice whole-grain bread, toasted
1 tablespoon cilantro leaves
2 tablespoons quark
2 tablespoons diced cucumber
Pinch sea salt

STEPS

1. Top toast with quark, cucumber, cilantro and sea salt.

2. Serve!

NUTRITION FACTS

Calories: 141 |Fat: 5 g|Carbohydrates: 13 g|Fiber: 2 g|Protein: 7 g|Sodium: 300 mg|Cholesterol: 20 mg

BANANA ENERGY BITES

SERVES FOR
16 PORTIONS

INGREDIENTS

1 overripe banana
1 cup dry quick-cooking rolled oats
1/2 cup roasted and salted pumpkin seeds (pepitas)
1/2 cup dried cranberries
1/2 cup natural peanut butter
1/4 cup miniature semisweet chocolate pieces

STEPS

1. In a bowl mash banana with a fork until smooth. Stir in oats; dried cranberries,

2. pumpkin seeds, peanut butter, and chocolate pieces. Using 1 tbsp. for each bite, shape into 32 balls; flatten slightly. Chill until ready to serve.

NUTRITION FACTS

Calories: 145 |Fat: 9 g|Carbohydrates: 13 g|Fiber: 1.6 g|Protein: 4.9 g|Sodium: 52 mg

COD IN FOIL

SERVES FOR
4 PEOPLE

INGREDIENTS

1 clove garlic, minced
1 red bell pepper, seeded and cubed
1 onion, minced
2 tomatoes, cubed
2 tablespoons olive oil
2 tablespoons chopped fresh basil
4 cod fillets
Aluminum foil
Lemon juice
Salt and ground black pepper to taste

STEPS

1. Preheat the oven to 425 degrees F.

2. Combine olive oil, onion, garlic

3. tomatoes, bell pepper, and basil, in a bowl and mix well.

4. Lay 4 sheets of aluminum foil on a work surface and place 1 cod fillet in the center of each. Spoon tomato mixture evenly on top of the 4 fillets. Sprinkle with lemon juice and season with salt and pepper. Place the second sheet of foil on top and seal the edges to make a parcel. Repeat with the remaining fillets and tomato mixture.

5. Bake in the preheated oven for about 18 minutes. Remove from the oven and carefully unwrap the parcels. Spoon onto warmed plates and serve immediately.

NUTRITION FACTS

Calories: 216 |Fat: 8 g|Carbohydrates: 10 g|Fiber: 3.3 g|Sodium: 146 mg |Protein: 27 g|Cholesterol: 51 mg

SPINACH SALMON CASSEROLE WITH CHEESE CREAM

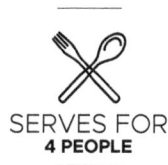

SERVES FOR
4 PEOPLE

INGREDIENTS

1/2 teaspoon red pepper flakes
1/2 teaspoon Italian seasoning
2 cup spinach, rinsed
2 tablespoons olive oil, divided
3 cloves garlic, minced
4 oz Mozzarella cheese, shredded
4 salmon fillets
8 oz cream cheese, softened

STEPS

1. Position a rack in the center of the oven and preheat the oven to 425 degrees F.

2. Add olive oil, garlic, Italian seasoning, and red pepper flakes into a bowl along with 1 teaspoon of salt and 1/2 teaspoon black pepper.

3. Arrange the salmon fillets in a baking dish and cover with the marinade, set aside for 10 minutes on the counter while prepping the other ingredients and the oven finishes preheating. Quickly wilt the spinach in a skillet with 1 tablespoon olive oil and set aside.

4. Sprinkle the softened cream cheese over the salmon fillets and lay spinach on top of the cream cheese. Finally, sprinkle mozzarella over the top.

5. Bake the spinach salmon casserole for 20 minutes.

6. Garnish with red chili pepper flakes and chopped parlsey. Serve!

NUTRITION FACTS

Calories: 927 |Fat: 58 g|Carbohydrates: 7.02 g|Sodium: 537 mg|Protein: 90 g|Cholesterol: 296 mg

CORNED BEEF

SERVES FOR
4 PEOPLE

INGREDIENTS

1 can beer
2 cups water
3 pounds corned beef brisket with spice packet
4 cloves garlic, minced

STEPS

1. Combine beer, water, and garlic in a multi-functional pressure cooker. Place trivet inside. Place brisket on the trivet and sprinkle spice packet on top.

2. Close and lock the lid. Select high pressure according to manufacturer's instructions; set timer for 95 minutes. Allow 10 minutes for pressure to build.

3. Release pressure carefully using the quick-release method according to manufacturer's instructions, about 6 minutes. Unlock and remove the lid.

4. Transfer brisket to a baking sheet, cover with aluminum foil and let rest for 10 minutes.

5. Serve!

NUTRITION FACTS

Calories: 416 |Fat: 28 g|Carbohydrates: 4.9 g|Protein: 27.7 g|Sodium: 1697 mg|Cholesterol: 146 mg

ITALIAN-STYLE TURKEY MEATBALLS

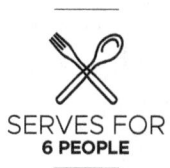

INGREDIENTS

1/8 teaspoon red pepper flake
1/2 cup shredded Parmesan cheese
1 pound ground turkey
1 cup crushed pork rinds
1 egg
1 tablespoon chopped fresh parsley
1 teaspoon minced garlic
1 teaspoon onion powder
1 teaspoon Italian seasoning
Aluminum foil
Cooking spray

STEPS

1. Line a baking sheet with aluminum foil and spray with cooking spray. Preheat the oven to 425 degrees F.

2. Combine pork rinds, ground turkey, garlic, onion powder, Parmesan cheese, egg, parsley, Italian seasoning, and red pepper flakes in a bowl. Mix with your hands until well combined.

3. Scoop out meat mixture to form twelve 1 1/2-inch meatballs. Place on the prepared baking sheet.

4. Bake in the preheated oven for 20 minutes.

5. Serve!

NUTRITION FACTS

Calories: 371 |Fat: 24 g|Carbohydrates: 1 g|Sodium: 426 mg|Protein: 40 g|Cholesterol: 146 mg

CHICKEN MARSALA

SERVES FOR
4 PEOPLE

INGREDIENTS

1/8 cup milk
1/4 cup chopped green onion
1/3 cup Marsala wine
1/3 cup heavy cream
1 cup sliced fresh mushrooms
4 skinless, boneless chicken breast halves
Salt and pepper to taste

STEPS

1. Heat oil in a skillet over medium heat. Add chicken and saute for 18 minutes.

2. Add green onion and mushrooms and saute until soft, then add Marsala wine and bring to a boil.

3. Boil for 3 minutes, seasoning with salt and pepper to taste. Stir in cream and milk and simmer until heated for about 6 minutes.

4. Serve!

NUTRITION FACTS

Calories: 241 |Fat: 9 g|Carbohydrate: 4.9 g|Protein: 28 g|Fiber: 0.4 g|Sodium: 90 mg|Cholesterol: 96 mg

SALMON PATTIES

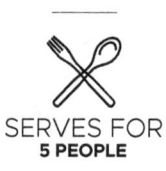

INGREDIENTS

1/4 cup chopped onion
1/2 cup seasoned dry bread crumbs
1 egg
1 tablespoon olive oil
15 ounces canned salmon

STEPS

1. Drain and reserve liquid from salmon. Mix onion, egg, bread crumbs, and salmon together.

2. Make into patties. If the mixture is too dry to form into patties, add reserved liquid from salmon.

3. In a frying pan, heat olive oil. Place patties in the pan. Cook each side, turning gently. Drain on paper towels and serve.

NUTRITION FACTS

Calories: 244 |Fat: 10 g|Carbohydrates: 9 g|Sodium: 522 mg|Fiber: 0.7 g|Protein: 23 g|Cholesterol: 73 mg

BRAISED CORNED BEEF BRISKET

INGREDIENTS

1 flat-cut corned beef brisket
1 tablespoon vegetable oil
1 onion, sliced
1 tablespoon browning sauce
2 tablespoons water
6 cloves garlic, sliced

STEPS

1. Preheat oven to 300 degrees F.

2. Discard any flavoring packet from corned beef. Brush brisket with browning sauce on both sides. Heat vegetable oil in a skillet over medium heat and brown brisket on both sides in the hot oil, for 7 minutes per side.

3. Place brisket on a rack set in a roasting pan. Add onion and garlic slices over brisket and add water to the roasting pan. Cover pan tightly with aluminum foil.

4. Roast in the preheated oven until meat is tender, about 5 hours.

5. Serve!

NUTRITION FACTS

Calories: 455 |Fat: 33 g|Carbohydrates: 5.4 g|Fiber: 0.7 g|Sodium: 1877 mg|Protein: 30 g|Cholesterol: 162 mg

BRISKET WITH BBQ SAUCE

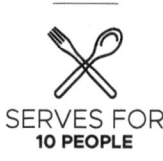

INGREDIENTS

1 cup sliced shallots, thinly sliced
1 bunch broccoli, cut into florets
1 1/2 tsp. olive oil
2 Tbsp. walnut pieces
Salt & freshly ground black pepper

STEPS

1. Preheat oven to 450 degrees F. Place walnuts on a pie plate and toast in the oven for 5 minutes. Transfer to a bowl and set aside.

2. In a nonstick skillet, heat oil over low heat. Add shallots and cook, stirring often, for about 12 minutes. Season with salt and pepper; set aside in the skillet.

3. Meanwhile, cook broccoli in boiling salted water for 5 minutes. Drain the broccoli and add it to the shallots in the skillet and toss to combine.

4. Transfer to a serving bowl and garnish with the toasted walnuts.

5. Serve!

NUTRITION FACTS

Calories: 113 |Fat: 4 g|Carbohydrates: 16 g|Protein: 7 g|Sodium: 51 mg|Cholesterol: 0 mg

SLOW COOKER BARBEQUE

INGREDIENTS

1 teaspoon garlic powder
1 teaspoon onion powder
1 (3 pounds) boneless chuck roast
18 ounces bottle barbeque sauce
Salt and pepper to taste

STEPS

1. Place roast into slow cooker. Sprinkle with onion powder and garlic powder, and season with salt and pepper. Pour barbeque sauce over meat. Cook on Low for 4 hours.

2. Remove meat from slow cooker, shred, and return to slow cooker. Cook for 1 more hour.

3. Serve!

NUTRITION FACTS

Calories: 344 |Fat: 17 g|Carbohydrate: 23 g|Sodium: 895 mg|Protein: 20 g|Fiber: 0.4 g|Cholesterol: 73 mg

BUFFALO PULLED CHICKEN

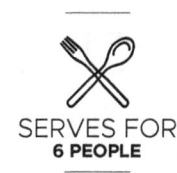

SERVES FOR
6 PEOPLE

INGREDIENTS

1/2 cup Buffalo wing sauce
1 celery ribs
2 tablespoons ranch salad dressing mix
4 boneless skinless chicken breast halves
crumbled blue cheese to taste

STEPS

1. In a 3-qt. slow cooker, mix wing sauce and 1/2 dressing mix. Add chicken. Cook, covered, on low, for about 3 hours.

2. Shred chicken with 2 forks. Garnish with blue cheese, and with remaining ranch dressing. Serve!

NUTRITION FACTS

Calories: 147 |Fat: 3 g|Carbohydrates: 6 g|Sodium: 1288 mg|Protein: 23 g|Cholesterol: 63 mg

CHICKEN WITH ONION AND CHEESY

INGREDIENTS

1/2 medium onion, sliced
1 cup shredded Colby-Monterey Jack cheese
1 medium green pepper, cut into strips
1 pound boneless skinless chicken breasts, cubed
2 teaspoons Mrs. Dash Garlic & Herb seasoning blend
2 tablespoons olive oil, divided

STEPS

1. Toss chicken with seasoning blend. In a nonstick skillet, heat 1 tablespoon oil over medium heat. Add chicken; cook and stir for 6 minutes. Remove from pan. In the same pan, add remaining oil, onion, and pepper; cook and stir for 4 minutes.

2. Stir in chicken; sprinkle with cheese. Remove from heat; let stand, covered, for about 5 minutes.

3. Serve!

NUTRITION FACTS

Calories: 293 |Fat: 17 g|Carbohydrates: 4 g|Sodium: 226 mg|Protein: 29 g|Cholesterol: 88 mg

MEXICAN-STYLE CHICKEN STRIPS

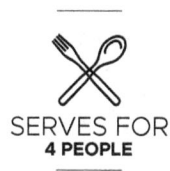

SERVES FOR
4 PEOPLE

INGREDIENTS

1/4 cup panko bread crumbs
1/4 cup dry bread crumbs
1/4 cup finely shredded Mexican cheese blend
1/4 cup butter, melted
1/2 cup finely crushed corn chips
1 pound chicken tenderloins
5 teaspoons taco seasoning
Dash cayenne pepper

STEPS

1. Preheat oven to 425 degrees F.

2. In a bowl mix the 1/2 cup finely crushed corn chips, 1/4 cup panko bread crumbs, 1/4 cup dry bread crumbs, 1/4 cup finely shredded Mexican cheese blend, 5 teaspoons taco seasoning, Dash cayenne pepper.

3. Place butter in a separate bowl. Dip chicken in butter, then roll in crumb mixture to coat; press to adhere. Place chicken on a foil-lined baking pan.

4. Bake for about 13 minutes, turning halfway through the cooking time.

5. Serve!

NUTRITION FACTS

Calories: 258 |Fat: 14 g|Carbohydrates: 7 g|Sodium: 351 mg|Protein: 28 g|Cholesterol: 85 mg

MEDITERRANEAN MEAT PIZZA

SERVES FOR
6 PEOPLE

INGREDIENTS

1/4 cup Greek olives
1/3 cup cherry tomatoes, halved
1/2 cup pizza sauce
1/2 cup drained water-packed artichoke hearts, chopped
1 large egg, lightly beaten
1 tablespoon Greek seasoning
1 cup shredded mozzarella cheese
1-1/2 pounds ground turkey
2 tablespoons crumbled feta cheese
2 tablespoons minced fresh basil

STEPS

1. Preheat oven to 425 degrees F.

2. In a bowl, combine turkey, egg, and Greek seasoning; mix. Press onto the bottom and 1-1/2-in. up sides of a greased 10-in. cast-iron ovenproof skillet.

3. Cook, without stirring, over medium heat until the bottom is no longer pink. Carefully drain drippings from the pan, leaving meat in the pan.

4. Bake for 10 minutes. Spread with pizza sauce; garnish with mozzarella, tomatoes, artichokes, olives, and feta.

5. Bake until cheese is melted, for 4 minutes longer. Cool 5 minutes before garnishing with basil.

NUTRITION FACTS

Calories: 272 |Fat: 15 g|Carbohydrates: 4 g|Fiber: 1 g| Sodium: 904 mg|Protein: 29 g|Cholesterol: 122 mg

CAULIFLOWER SOUP

SERVES FOR
8 PEOPLE

INGREDIENTS

1/8 teaspoon pepper
1/4 cup chopped celery
1/2 to 1 teaspoon hot pepper sauce
1 cup shredded cheddar cheese
1 medium head cauliflower, broken into florets
1 medium carrot, shredded
2 teaspoons chicken bouillon
2 cups 2% milk
2-1/2 cups water
3 tablespoons butter
3 tablespoons all-purpose flour
3/4 teaspoon salt

STEPS

1. In a Dutch oven, combine the cauliflower, celery, carrot, water, and bouillon. Bring to a boil. Reduce heat; cover and simmer for 15 minutes.

2. In a saucepan, melt butter. Stir in the flour, salt, and pepper until smooth. Gradually add milk. Bring to a boil over medium heat; cook and stir for 2 minutes. Reduce heat. Stir in the cheese until melted, adding hot pepper sauce. Stir into the cauliflower mixture.

3. Serve!

NUTRITION FACTS

Calories: 159 |Fat: 11 g|Carbohydrates: 10 g|Fiber: 2 g|Sodium: 617 mg|Protein: 7 g|Cholesterol: 35 mg

CHICKEN TACO SALAD

INGREDIENTS

1/4 teaspoon dried oregano
1/4 teaspoon crushed red pepper flakes
1/2 teaspoon each white pepper, ground chipotle pepper, and paprika
1 teaspoon each ground cumin, seasoned salt, and pepper
1 cup chicken broth
1-1/2 pounds boneless skinless chicken breasts
3 teaspoons chili powder
9 cups torn romaine
Sliced avocado
Shredded cheddar cheese
Chopped tomato
Sliced green onions, and salad dressing of choice

STEPS

1. In a bowl mix the 3 teaspoons chili powder, 1 teaspoon each ground cumin, seasoned salt, and pepper, 1/2 teaspoon each white pepper, ground chipotle pepper, and paprika, 1/4 teaspoon dried oregano, 1/4 teaspoon crushed red pepper flakes, and put over the chicken; mix. Place in a 3-qt. slow cooker. Add broth. Cook, covered, on low 3 hours.

2. Remove chicken; cool slightly. Shred chicken with 2 forks.

3. Serve with sliced avocado, cheddar cheese, chopped tomato, green onions, and salad dressing desired.

NUTRITION FACTS

Calories: 143 |Fat: 3 g|Carbohydrates: 4 g|Fiber: 2 g|Sodium: 516 mg|Protein: 24 g|Cholesterol: 63 mg

ASPARAGUS-MUSHROOM FRITTATA

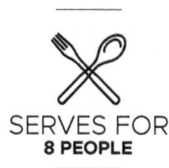

INGREDIENTS

1/4 cup sliced baby portobello mushrooms
1/4 teaspoon pepper
1/2 teaspoon salt
1/2 cup whole-milk ricotta cheese
1/2 cup finely chopped sweet red
1 tablespoon olive oil
1 large onion, halved and thinly sliced
2 tablespoons lemon juice
8 large eggs
8 ounces frozen asparagus spears, thawed

STEPS

1. Preheat oven to 375 degrees F.

2. In a bowl, whisk eggs, lemon juice, ricotta cheese, salt, and pepper. In a 10-in. ovenproof skillet, heat oil over medium heat. Add onion, asparagus, red pepper, and mushrooms; cook and stir for 7 minutes.

3. Remove from heat; remove asparagus from skillet. Reserve eight spears; cut remaining asparagus into 2-in. pieces. Return cut asparagus to skillet; stir in egg mixture. Arrange reserved asparagus spears over eggs. Bake, uncovered, for about 23 minutes. Let stand 2 minutes. Cut into wedges.

4. Serve!

NUTRITION FACTS

Calories: 130 |Fat: 8 g|Carbohydrates: 5 g|Protein: 9 g|Sodium: 240 mg|Fiber: 1 g|Cholesterol: 192 mg

CHICKEN WITH BACON AND CAPRESE

SERVES FOR
4 PEOPLE

INGREDIENTS

1/4 teaspoon pepper
1/2 teaspoon salt
1 tablespoon olive oil
2 plum tomatoes, sliced
4 slices part-skim mozzarella cheese
4 boneless skinless chicken breast halves
6 fresh basil leaves, thinly sliced
8 bacon strips

STEPS

1. Preheat oven to 400 degrees F. Place bacon in an ungreased 15x10x1-in. baking pan. Bake until partially cooked but not crisp, for 7 minutes. Remove to paper towels to drain.

2. Place chicken in an ungreased 13x9-in. baking pan; brush with oil and sprinkle with salt and pepper.

3. Top with tomatoes and basil. Wrap each in 2 bacon strips, arranging bacon in a crisscross.

4. Bake, uncovered for 20 minutes. Garnish with cheese; bake until melted, 1 minute longer.

5. Serve!

NUTRITION FACTS

Calories: 373 |Fat: 18 g|Carbohydrates: 3 g|Fiber: 0 g|Protein: 47 g|Sodium: 821 mg|Cholesterol: 123 mg

GREEK SALAD

SERVES FOR
8 PEOPLE

INGREDIENTS

1/8 teaspoon pepper
1/4 teaspoon dried oregano
1/4 cup olive oil
1/4 teaspoon salt
3/4 cup pitted Greek olives
3/4 cup crumbled feta cheese
1 small red onion, halved and thinly sliced
2-1/2 cups thinly sliced English cucumbers
3 tablespoons red wine vinegar
4 large tomatoes, seeded and coarsely chopped

STEPS

1. In a bowl, whisk vinegar, oil, oregano, salt, and pepper, until blended.

2. In a bowl salad place tomatoes, onion, and cucumbers. Add the prepared sauce. Sprinkle over salad.

3. Garnish with olives and cheese.

4. Serve!

NUTRITION FACTS

Calories: 148 |Fat: 12 g|Carbohydrates: 7 g|Fiber: 2 g|Protein: 3 g|Sodium: 389 mg|Cholesterol: 6 mg

ALMOND CHICKEN SALAD

SERVES FOR
8 PEOPLE

INGREDIENTS

1/8 teaspoon ground mustard
1/8 teaspoon paprika
1/4 teaspoon onion powder
1/4 teaspoon celery salt
1/4 cup sour cream
1/2 teaspoon pepper
1/2 cup slivered almonds, toasted
1/2 cup Miracle Whip
3/4 cup sliced green onions
1 tablespoon prepared mustard
1 teaspoon salt
1 kiwifruit, peeled and sliced
1 cup chopped celery
1-1/2 cups seedless green grapes, halved
3 hard-boiled large eggs, chopped
4 cups cubed cooked chicken

STEPS

1. In a bowl, combine chicken, celery, onions, grapes, and eggs.

2. In another bowl, combine the Miracle Whip, sour cream, mustard, salt, pepper, onion powder, celery salt, ground mustard, paprika; stir until smooth.

3. Pour over the chicken mixture and toss gently. Add the almonds and serve immediately.

4. Garnish with kiwi sliced.

NUTRITION FACTS

Calories: 351 |Fat: 23 g|Carbohydrates: 10 g|Fiber: 2 g|Sodium: 540 mg|Protein: 25 g|Cholesterol: 152 mg

VEGETABLE, STEAK AND EGGS

SERVES FOR
4 PEOPLE

INGREDIENTS

1/4 cup shredded Parmesan cheese
1/4 teaspoon pepper
1/2 teaspoon salt
1 beef skirt steak
1 teaspoon Montreal steak seasoning
1 medium zucchini, halved lengthwise
and cut into 1/4-inch slices
1 medium yellow summer squash, halved
lengthwise and cut into 1/4-inch slices
1 medium sweet red pepper, chopped
2 tablespoons butter, divided
4 large eggs
5 ounces fresh baby spinach

STEPS

1. Rub steak with seasoning.

2. Grill steak, covered, over medium-high heat for 5 minutes on each side. Let stand 5 minutes.

3. Meanwhile, in a nonstick skillet, heat 1 tablespoon butter over medium heat. Saute zucchini, red pepper, and squash, for 8 minutes. Add spinach, salt, and pepper; cook and stir until wilted, 2 minutes. Divide among 4 plates; keep warm.

4. In the same skillet, heat the remaining butter. Break eggs, 1 at a time, into pan; reduce heat to low. Cook to desired doneness. Thinly slice steak across the grain; serve over vegetables.

5. Garnish with egg and cheese. Serve!

NUTRITION FACTS

Calories: 344 |Fat: 21 g|Carbohydrates: 7 g|Fiber: 2 g|Sodium: 770 mg|Protein: 33 g|Cholesetrol: 259 mg

POACHED SALMON

SERVES FOR
8 PEOPLE

INGREDIENTS

1/2 cup dry white wine
1 bay leaf
1 salmon fillet
1 medium onion, chopped
1 tablespoon soy sauce
2 celery ribs, chopped
4 sprigs fresh parsley
6 cups water
8 whole peppercorns
Lemon slices and fresh dill

STEPS

1. In a saucepan, combine the water, onion chopped, celery ribs chopped, sprigs fresh parsley, dry white wine, soy sauce, whole peppercorns, bay leaf. Bring to a boil; reduce heat. Simmer, covered, 35 minutes. Strain, discarding vegetables and spices.

2. Cut three 20x3-in. strips of heavy-duty foil; crisscross so they resemble spokes of a wheel. Place strips on the bottom and up sides of a 7-qt. oval slow cooker. Pour poaching liquid into slow cooker. Carefully add salmon.

3. Cook, covered, on high for 65 minutes. Using the foil strips as handles, remove salmon from cooking liquid.

4. Serve warm or cold, with lemon and dill.

NUTRITION FACTS

Calories: 266 |Fat: 16 g|Carbohydrates: 0 g|Fiber: 0 g|Protein: 29 g|Sodium: 97 mg|Cholesterol: 85 mg

ITALIAN-STYLE ALMOND VEGETABLE STIR-FRY

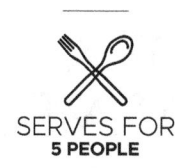

SERVES FOR
5 PEOPLE

INGREDIENTS

1/4 cup slivered almonds, toasted
1 large sweet red pepper, cut into 1-inch chunks
1 tablespoon minced fresh gingerroot
1 teaspoon sesame oil
1 small onion, cut into thin wedges
1 teaspoon cornstarch
1 teaspoon sugar
2 tablespoons reduced-sodium soy sauce
2 tablespoons canola oil
2 garlic cloves, minced
3 tablespoons cold water
4 cups fresh broccoli florets

STEPS

1. In a bowl, combine cornstarch and sugar. Stir in water, soy sauce, and sesame oil until smooth; set aside.

2. In a nonstick wok, stir-fry broccoli in hot oil for 3 minutes. Add onion, garlic pepper, and ginger; stir-fry for 3 minutes. Reduce heat. Stir soy sauce mixture; stir into vegetables with nuts. Cook and stir for 3 minutes.

3. Serve!

NUTRITION FACTS

Calories: 143 |Fat: 10 g|Carbohydrates: 11 g|Fiber: 3 g|Protein: 4 g|Sodium: 260 mg|Cholesterol: 0 mg

PORK CHOPS WITH PARMESAN SAUCE

SERVES FOR
4 PEOPLE

INGREDIENTS

1/4 teaspoon pepper
1/4 teaspoon dried thyme
1/4 teaspoon ground nutmeg
1/3 cup grated Parmesan cheese
1/2 teaspoon salt
1 cup fat-free milk
1 tablespoon butter
2 tablespoons all-purpose flour
2 tablespoons grated onion
3 teaspoons minced fresh parsley
4 boneless pork loin chops

STEPS

1. Sprinkle pork chops with salt and pepper.

2. In a nonstick skillet, cook chops in butter over medium heat until meat juices run clear; remove and keep warm.

3. Combine flour and milk until smooth; stir into pan. Bring to a boil; cook and stir for 3 minutes. Add the Parmesan cheese, thyme, onion, and prasley; heat through.

4. Serve with chops.

NUTRITION FACTS

Calories: 244 |Fat: 11 g|Carbohydrates: 7 g|Fiber: 0 g|Protein: 27 g|Sodium: 475 mg|Cholesterol: 69 mg

CHEESY CREAM OF ASPARAGUS SOUP

SERVES FOR
6 PEOPLE

INGREDIENTS

1/4 cup butter
1 cup shredded Monterey Jack cheese
1-1/2 teaspoons salt
2 tablespoons all-purpose flour
3/4 to 1 teaspoon pepper
4 cups whole milk
4 to 5 drops hot pepper sauce
12 ounces each frozen cut asparagus
Roasted asparagus tips

STEPS

1. Prepare asparagus according to package directions; drain and set aside. In a saucepan, melt butter. Stir in flour until smooth; gradually add milk. Bring to a boil; cook and stir until thickened, about 3 minutes. Cool slightly.

2. Pour half the milk mixture into a blender; add half the asparagus.

3. Cover and process until very smooth; return soup to the saucepan. Repeat with the remaining milk mixture and asparagus. Stir in the cheese, hot pepper sauce, salt, and pepper; heat through.

4. Garnish with roasted asparagus tips.

5. Serve!

NUTRITION FACTS

Calories: 261 |Fat: 19 g|Carbohydrates: 12 g|Protein: 12 g|Sodium: 852 mg|Fiber: 1 g|Cholesterol: 59 mg

HAM SALAD

SERVES FOR
10 PEOPLE

INGREDIENTS

3/4 cup mayonnaise
1/4 cup sliced green onions
1/3 cup chopped pecans and almonds,
toasted
1/2 teaspoon Worcestershire sauce
1/2 teaspoon seasoned salt
1/2 cup finely chopped celery
1 tablespoon honey
2 tablespoons minced fresh chives
2 teaspoons spicy brown mustard
5 cups diced fully cooked ham
Slider buns, split

STEPS

1. Mix the mayonnaise, celery,

2. green onions, fresh chives, honey, spicy brown mustard,

3. Worcestershire sauce, seasoned salt. Stir in ham. Refrigerate, covered, until serving.

4. Stir in pecans before serving.

5. Serve on buns.

NUTRITION FACTS

Calories: 254 |Fat: 20 g|Carbohydrates: 4 g|Fiber: 1 g|Protein: 16 g|Sodium: 1023 mg|Cholesterol: 43 mg

SHRIMP GAZPACHO

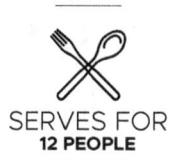

INGREDIENTS

1/4 teaspoon hot pepper sauce
1/2 cup lime juice
1/2 cup minced fresh cilantro
1/2 teaspoon salt
1 pound peeled and deveined cooked shrimp (31-40 per pound), tails removed
1 medium cucumber, seeded and diced
2 cups cold water
2 medium tomatoes, seeded and chopped
2 medium ripe avocados, peeled and chopped
6 cups spicy hot V8 juice

STEPS

1. In a nonreactive bowl, mix the spicy hot V8 juice, cold water, lime juice, fresh cilantro, salt, hot pepper sauce.

2. Gently stir the shrimp, cucumber, tomatoes, and avocados.

3. Refrigerate, covered, 1 hour before serving.

NUTRITION FACTS

Calories: 112 |Fat: 4 g|Carbohydrates: 9 g|Sodium: 399 mg|Fiber: 3 g|Protein: 10 g|Cholesterol: 57 mg

SAUSAGE SALAD LETTUCE WRAPS

INGREDIENTS

3/4 cup ranch salad dressing
1/4 cup watercress, chopped
1/3 cup crumbled blue cheese
1 medium tomato, chopped
1 medium ripe avocado, peeled and diced
1 pound bulk pork sausage
2 tablespoons minced fresh chives
4 hard-boiled large eggs, chopped
6 large iceberg lettuce leaves, edges trimmed

STEPS

1. Mix dressing, blue cheese, and watercress.

2. In a skillet, cook and crumble sausage over medium heat, for 8 minutes; drain. Stir in chives.

3. To serve, spoon sausage into lettuce leaves.

4. Garnish with avocado, eggs, and tomato.

5. Sprinkle with dressing mixture.

6. Serve!

NUTRITION FACTS

Calories: 433 |Fat: 38 g|Carbohydrates: 7 g|Fiber: 3 g|Protein: 15 g|Sodium: 887 mg|Cholesterol: 174 mg

CHICKEN THIGHS WITH SHALLOTS & SPINACH

SERVES FOR
6 PEOPLE

INGREDIENTS

1/4 teaspoon salt
1/4 cup reduced-fat sour cream
1/3 cup white wine
1/2 teaspoon seasoned salt
1/2 teaspoon pepper
1-1/2 teaspoons olive oil
4 shallots, thinly sliced
6 boneless skinless chicken thighs
10 ounces fresh spinach, trimmed

STEPS

1. Sprinkle chicken with seasoned salt and pepper.

2. In a nonstick skillet, heat oil over medium heat. Add chicken; cook for about 7 minutes on each side. Remove from pan; keep warm.

3. In the same pan, cook and stir shallots until tender. Add wine; bring to a boil. Cook until wine is reduced by half.

4. Add spinach and salt; cook and stir just until spinach is wilted.

5. Stir in sour cream; serve with chicken.

NUTRITION FACTS

Calories: 223 |Fat: 10 g|Carbohydrates: 7 g|Fiber: 1 g|Protein: 23 g|Sodium: 360 mg|Cholesterol: 77 mg

CRUNCHY CHILI LIME SHRIMP

INGREDIENTS

1/4 cup chopped fresh cilantro
1/4 cup olive oil
1/4 teaspoon pepper
1/2 teaspoon salt
1 teaspoon paprika
1 teaspoon ground ancho chili pepper
1 teaspoon ground cumin
1 medium lime
1 cup crushed tortilla chips
1 cup cherry tomatoes, halved
1 medium ripe avocado, peeled and cubed
2 pounds uncooked shrimp (26-30 per pound), peeled and deveined
4 garlic cloves, minced

STEPS

1. Preheat oven to 400 degrees F. Place the shrimp, garlic, paprika, chili pepper, cumin, salt, and pepper, in a greased 15x10x1-in. pan. Finely grate the zest from the lime. Cut lime crosswise in half; squeeze the juice. Add zest and juice to shrimp mixture; toss to coat.

2. In a bowl, combine crushed chips, cilantro, and oil; sprinkle over shrimp mixture. Bake until shrimp turn pink, for about 14 minutes.

3. Garnish with tomatoes and avocado.

4. Serve!

NUTRITION FACTS

Calories: 230 |Fat: 13 g|Carbohydrates: 10 g|Fiber: 2 g|Protein: 20 g|Sodium: 315 mg|Cholesterol: 138 mg

PORTOBELLO MUSHROOMS FLORENTINE

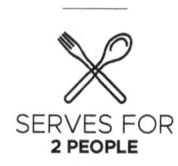
INGREDIENTS

1/8 teaspoon garlic salt
1/8 teaspoon pepper
1/8 teaspoon salt
1/4 cup crumbled goat
1/2 teaspoon olive oil
1 small onion, chopped
1 cup fresh baby spinach
2 large eggs
2 large portobello mushrooms, stems removed
Cooking spray
Minced fresh basil

STEPS

1. Preheat oven to 425 degrees F. Sprinkle the mushrooms with the cooking spray; place in a pan, stem side up.

2. Drizzle with garlic salt and pepper. Bake, uncovered, for about 10 minutes.

3. Meanwhile, in a nonstick skillet, heat oil over medium heat; saute onion until tender. Stir in spinach until wilted.

4. Whisk together eggs and salt; add to skillet. Cook and stir until eggs are thickened and no liquid egg remains; spoon onto mushrooms.

5. Garnish with cheese and basil.

6. Serve!

NUTRITION FACTS

Calories: 126 |Fat: 5 g|Carbohydrates: 10 g|Fiber: 3 g|Protein: 11 g|Sodium: 472 mg|Cholesterol: 18 mg

PORK SALAD

INGREDIENTS

1/2 teaspoon ground cumin
1/2 teaspoon dried oregano
1 teaspoon chili powder
1 teaspoon pepper
1 small red onion, chopped
1 cup fresh corn
1 cup crumbled shredded part-skim
mozzarella cheese
1 boneless pork loin roast
1-1/2 cups apple cider
1-1/2 teaspoons salt
1-1/2 teaspoons hot pepper sauce
2 medium tomatoes, chopped
3 garlic cloves, minced
4 ounces chopped green chiles, drained
12 cups torn mixed salad greens
15 ounces black beans, rinsed and
drained
Salad dressing of your choice

STEPS

1. Place pork in a 5-qt. slow cooker. In a bowl, mix green chiles, chili powder, cider, garlic, salt, pepper sauce, pepper, cumin, and oregano; pour over pork. Cook, covered, on low 5 hours.

2. Remove roast from slow cooker; discard cooking juices. Shred pork with 2 forks. Arrange salad greens on a large serving platter.

3. Top with pork, onion, black beans, tomatoes, corn, and cheese.

4. Serve with salad dressing.

NUTRITION FACTS

Calories: 233 |Fat: 8 g|Carbohydrates: 12 g|Fiber: 3 g|Protein: 28 g|Sodium: 321 mg|Cholesterol: 67 mg

GRILLED BUTTERMILK CHICKEN

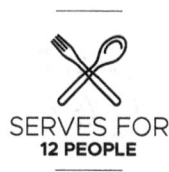

INGREDIENTS

1/2 teaspoon salt
1-1/2 cups buttermilk
4 fresh thyme sprigs
4 garlic cloves, halved
12 boneless skinless chicken breast halves

STEPS

1. Place the buttermilk, garlic, thyme, and salt in a bowl. Add chicken and turn to coat. Refrigerate for 10 hours, turning occasionally.

2. Drain chicken, discarding marinade. Grill, covered, over medium heat for about 8 minutes per side.

3. Serve!

NUTRITION FACTS

Calories: 189 |Fat: 4 g|Carbohydrates: 1 g|Fiber: 0 g|Protein: 35 g|Sodium: 168 mg|Cholesterol: 95 mg

GRILLED VEGETABLE SALAD

SERVES FOR
2 PEOPLE

INGREDIENTS

1/4 teaspoon ground mustard
1/2 teaspoon grated onion
1/2 teaspoon poppy seeds
1 tablespoon cider vinegar
2 tablespoons canola oil
2 teaspoons sugar
Dash salt
SALAD:
1/8 teaspoon freshly ground pepper
1/4 teaspoon salt
1 small zucchini, cut into 3/4-inch pieces
1 small sweet yellow pepper, cut into
1-inch pieces
1 teaspoon minced fresh thyme
2 teaspoons olive oil
2 teaspoons minced fresh basil
2 teaspoons minced fresh parsley
2/3 cup cherry tomatoes

STEPS

1. In a bowl, whisk the canola oil, cider vinegar, sugar, onion, poppy seeds, ground mustard, and salt until blended. Refrigerate until serving.

2. In another bowl, combine zucchini, yellow pepper, and tomatoes. Add oil, salt, and pepper; toss to coat. Transfer to a grill wok; place on grill rack. Grill, covered, over medium heat for 13 minutes, stirring occasionally.

3. Transfer vegetables to a serving bowl; sprinkle with herbs.

4. Serve with dressing.

NUTRITION FACTS

Calories: 219 |Fat: 19 g|Carbohydrates: 11 g|Fiber: 2 g|Protein: 2 g|Sodium: 378 mg|Cholesterol: 0 mg

ITALIAN SAUSAGE AND PROVOLONE SKEWERS

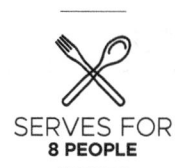

INGREDIENTS

1/4 teaspoon salt
1/2 teaspoon pepper
1 tablespoon olive oil
1 large onion
1 large sweet red pepper
1 large green pepper
2 cups cherry tomatoes
12 ounces fully cooked Italian chicken sausage links, cut into 1-1/4-inch slices
16 cubes provolone cheese (3/4 inch each)

STEPS

1. Cut onion and peppers into 1-in. pieces; place in a bowl. Add oil, tomatoes, salt, and pepper; toss to coat.

2. On 16 metal or soaked wooden skewers, alternately thread sausage and vegetables.

3. Grill, covered, over medium heat for 12 minutes, turning occasionally.

4. Remove kabobs from grill; thread one cheese cube onto each kabob.

5. Serve!

NUTRITION FACTS

Calories: 220 |Fat: 13 g|Carbohydrates: 7 g|Fiber: 2 g|Protein: 20 g|Sodium: 682 mg|Cholesterol: 75 mg

COLORFUL FRITTATA

**SERVES FOR
6 PEOPLE**

INGREDIENTS

1/4 teaspoon pepper
1/4 cup shredded Parmesan cheese
1/4 cup crumbled feta cheese
1/2 teaspoon salt
1 garlic clove, minced
1 cup fat-free milk
1 small yellow summer squash, thinly sliced
1 small zucchini, thinly sliced
1 small onion, chopped
1 cup shredded part-skim mozzarella cheese
1 medium tomato, sliced
2 tablespoons minced fresh basil
4 large eggs

STEPS

1. In a microwave-safe bowl, combine the zucchini, squash, and onion. Cover and microwave on high for 8 minutes; drain well.

2. Transfer to a 9-in. pie plate coated with cooking spray. Garnish with mozzarella, tomato, and feta cheese.

3. In a bowl, whisk the eggs, milk, garlic, basil, salt, and pepper; pour over the cheese and tomato layer.

4. Sprinkle with Parmesan cheese.

5. Bake, uncovered, at 400 degrees F for about 50 minutes.

6. Let stand for 5 minutes before serving.

NUTRITION FACTS

Calories: 161 |Fat: 9 g|Carbohydrates: 7 g|Fiber: 1 g|Protein: 13 g|Sodium: 494 mg|Cholesterol: 142 mg

CHICKEN STRIPS WITH PANKO

SERVES FOR
4 PEOPLE

INGREDIENTS

1/4 teaspoon crushed red pepper flakes
1/4 cup butter, cubed
1/2 teaspoon salt
1/2 cup panko bread crumbs
1/2 cup grated Parmesan cheese
1 day-old everything bagel, torn
1 pound chicken tenderloins

STEPS

1. Preheat oven to 450 degrees F. Pulse torn bagel in a food processor until coarse crumbs form. Place 1/2 cup bagel crumbs in a bowl; toss with panko, cheese, and pepper flakes.

2. In a microwave-safe bowl, microwave put the butter until melted. Sprinkle chicken with salt. Dip in warm butter, then coat with crumb mixture, patting to help adhere.

3. Place on a greased rack in a 15x10x1- in. pan.

4. Bake for 16 minutes.

5. Serve!

NUTRITION FACTS

Calories: 243 |Fat: 12 g|Carbohydrates: 6 g|Fiber: 0 g|Protein: 30 g|Sodium: 593 mg|Cholesterol: 85 mg

CHICKEN NUGGETS

INGREDIENTS

1/4 cup canola oil
1/2 teaspoon pepper
1 teaspoon poultry seasoning
1 teaspoon ground mustard
1 teaspoon paprika
1 cup all-purpose flour
2 pounds boneless skinless chicken breasts
4 teaspoons seasoned salt

STEPS

1. In a shallow dish, combine the flour, seasoned salt, poultry seasoning, ground mustard, paprika, and pepper. Flatten chicken to 1/2-in. thickness, then cut into 1-1/2-in. pieces. Add chicken, a few pieces at a time, to the dish and turn to coat.

2. In a skillet, cook chicken in oil in batches for about 8 minutes.

3. Serve!

NUTRITION FACTS

Calories: 212 |Fat: 10 g|Carbohydrates: 6 g|Fiber: 0 g|Protein: 24 g|Sodium: 435 mg|Cholesterol: 63 mg

APPLE AND POMEGRANATE SALAD

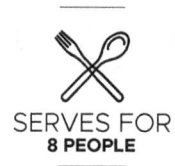

SERVES FOR
8 PEOPLE

INGREDIENTS

1/4 teaspoon salt
1/4 cup olive oil
1/4 cup white wine vinegar
1/2 cup pomegranate seeds
1/2 cup chopped pecans, toasted
1/2 cup shredded Parmesan cheese
1 large apple, chopped
1 tablespoon lemon juice
2 tablespoons sugar
8 cups romaine, torn

STEPS

1. In a bowl, combine romaine, pecans, pomegranate seeds, and cheese. Toss apple with lemon juice and add to salad.

2. In another bowl, whisk the oil, white wine vinegar, lemon juice, and sugar, until blended. Sprinkle over salad; toss to coat.

3. Serve immediately!

NUTRITION FACTS

Calories: 165 |Fat: 13 g|Carbohydrates: 10 g|Fiber: 2 g|Protein: 3 g|Sodium: 163 mg|Cholesterol: 4 mg

MUSHROOM SOUP

SERVES FOR
6 PEOPLE

INGREDIENTS

1/8 teaspoon pepper
1/4 cup chopped onion
1/2 teaspoon salt
1/2 pound sliced fresh mushrooms
1 cup half-and-half cream
2 tablespoons butter
6 tablespoons all-purpose flour
14-1/2 ounces chicken broth

STEPS

1. In a saucepan, heat butter over medium heat; saute onion, and mushrooms until tender.

2. Mix flour, salt, pepper, and 1 can broth until smooth; stir into mushroom mixture. Stir in the remaining can of broth. Bring to a boil; cook and stir until thickened, about 2 minutes. Reduce heat; stir in cream. Simmer, uncovered, until flavors are blended, about 16 minutes, stirring occasionally.

3. Serve!

NUTRITION FACTS

Calories: 136 |Fat: 8 g|Carbohydrates: 10 g|Fiber: 1 g|Protein: 4 g|Sodium: 842 mg|Cholesterol: 33 mg

BURGER WRAPS

SERVES FOR
4 PEOPLE

INGREDIENTS

1/4 cup chopped red onion
1/4 teaspoon pepper
1/3 cup crumbled feta cheese
1/2 medium ripe avocado, peeled and
cut into 8 slices
1/2 teaspoon salt
1 pound lean ground beef (90% lean)
8 Bibb lettuce leaves
2 tablespoons Miracle Whip Light
Chopped cherry tomatoes

STEPS

1. In a bowl, combine beef, salt, and pepper, mixing lightly but thoroughly. Shape into eight 1/2-in.-thick patties.

2. Grill burgers, covered, over medium heat for 4 minutes on each side. Place burgers in lettuce leaves. Combine feta and Miracle Whip; spread over burgers. Garnish with red onion, avocado, and tomatoes.

3. Serve!

NUTRITION FACTS

Calories: 252 |Fat: 15 g|Carbohydrates: 5 g|Fiber: 2 g|Protein: 24 g|Sodium: 518 mg|Cholesterol: 78 mg

SHAKSHUKA

INGREDIENTS

1/2 to 1 teaspoon chili powder
1/2 teaspoon salt
1 medium onion, chopped
1 garlic clove, minced
1 teaspoon ground cumin
1 teaspoon pepper
1 teaspoon Sriracha chili sauce
2 tablespoons olive oil
2 medium tomatoes, chopped
4 large eggs
Chopped fresh cilantro
Whole pita breads, toasted

STEPS

1. In a cast-iron skillet, heat oil over medium heat. Add onion; cook and stir until tender, for 5 minutes. Add garlic, seasonings and, chili sauce; cook 30 seconds longer. Add tomatoes; cook until mixture is thickened, stirring occasionally, for 5 minutes.

2. With the back of a spoon, make 4 wells in the vegetable mixture; break an egg into each well. Cook, covered until egg whites are completely set and yolks begin to thicken but are not hard, for 5 minutes.

3. Garnish with cilantro.

4. Serve with pita bread.

NUTRITION FACTS

Calories: 159 |Fat: 12 g|Carbohydrates: 6 g|Fiber: 2 g|Protein: 7 g|Sodium: 381 mg|Cholesterol: 186 mg

CREAM OF CAULIFLOWER SOUP

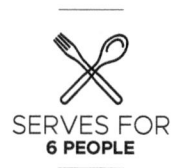

SERVES FOR
6 PEOPLE

INGREDIENTS

1/3 cup thinly sliced green onions
1/2 teaspoon salt
1 tablespoon minced chives
1-1/2 cups shredded reduced-fat
cheddar cheese
2 tablespoons butter
2 tablespoons all-purpose flour
2 cups chicken broth
2 cups 1% milk
2 tablespoons dry sherry
2-1/4 cups frozen cauliflower, thawed
and chopped

STEPS

1. In a saucepan, saute onions in butter until tender.

2. Stir in flour and salt until blended. Gradually add broth. Bring to a boil; cook and stir for 3 minutes. Reduce heat.

3. Add cauliflower; simmer for 2 minutes. Add the milk and cheese; cook and stir until cheese is melted. Stir in sherry.

4. Garnish with chives.

5. Serve!

NUTRITION FACTS

Calories: 186 |Fat: 11 g|Carbohydrates: 10 g|Fiber: 1 g|Protein: 13 g|Sodium: 792 mg|Cholesterol: 36 mg

SPEEDY SALMON PATTIES

SERVES FOR
3 PEOPLE

INGREDIENTS

1/8 teaspoon pepper
1/4 teaspoon salt
1/3 cup finely chopped onion
1/2 teaspoon Worcestershire sauce
1 large egg, beaten
2 teaspoons butter
5 saltines, crushed
14-3/4 ounces salmon, drained, bones
and skin removed

STEPS

1. In a bowl, combine the onion, egg, saltines crushed, Worcestershire sauce, salt, and pepper. Crumble salmon over mixture and mix well. Shape into 6 patties.

2. In a skillet over medium heat, fry patties in butter for 4 minutes on each side.

3. Serve!

NUTRITION FACTS

Calories: 288 |Fat: 15 g|Carbohydrates: 5 g|Fiber: 0 g|Protein: 31 g|Sodium: 1063 mg|Cholesterol: 139 mg

MEXICAN-STYLE STUFFED ZUCCHINI

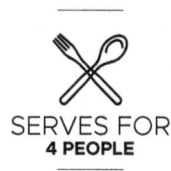

SERVES FOR
4 PEOPLE

INGREDIENTS

1/8 teaspoon pepper
1/4 teaspoon salt
1 pound ground beef
1 garlic clove, minced
1 cup shredded Havarti cheese with jalapeno
2 large zucchini
2 tablespoons minced fresh basil
3/4 cup crumbled feta cheese, divided

STEPS

1. Cut each zucchini in half lengthwise; cut a thin slice from the bottoms so they sit flat. Scoop out pulp, leaving 1/4-in. shells. Place zucchini shells in a microwave- and oven-safe dish. Cover and microwave on high for 4 minutes; drain and set aside.

2. In a cast-iron skillet over medium heat, cook beef and garlic; drain. Stir in the Havarti cheese, 1/2 cup feta cheese, basil, salt, and pepper.

3. Fill zucchini with meat mixture. Bake at 425 degrees F for about 16 minutes.

4. Garnish with remaining feta; bake 6 minutes longer.

5. Serve!

NUTRITION FACTS

Calories: 391 |Fat: 25 g|Carbohydrates: 7 g|Fiber: 3 g|Protein: 32 g|Sodium: 588 mg|Cholesterol: 108 mg

TOMATO WALNUT TILAPIA

INGREDIENTS

1/4 teaspoon salt
1/4 teaspoon pepper
1 tablespoon butter
1 medium tomato, thinly sliced
4 tilapia fillets
TOPPING:
1/4 cup chopped walnuts
1/2 cup soft bread crumbs
1-1/2 teaspoons butter, melted
2 tablespoons lemon juice

STEPS

1. Sprinkle fillets with salt and pepper. In a skillet coated with cooking spray, cook fillets in butter over medium heat until lightly browned, for 4 minutes on each side.

2. Transfer fish to a broiler pan; garnish with tomato. Combine the walnuts, bread crumbs, butter, and lemon juice; spoon over the tomato slices.

3. Broil 3-4 in. from the heat for about 3 minutes.

4. Serve!

NUTRITION FACTS

Calories: 202 |Fat: 10 g|Carbohydrates: 6 g|Fiber: 1 g|Protein: 23 g|Sodium: 251 mg|Cholesterol: 67 mg

COLORFUL VEGGIE SALAD

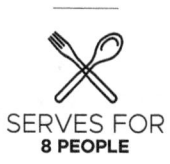

SERVES FOR
8 PEOPLE

INGREDIENTS

1/8 teaspoon garlic salt
1/4 cup each chopped sweet yellow,
orange and red pepper
1/4 cup thinly sliced red onion
1/2 English cucumber, cut lengthwise in
half and sliced
1 celery rib, thinly sliced
1 cup each red and yellow cherry
tomatoes, halved
2 medium carrots, thinly sliced
2/3 cup Pesto Buttermilk Dressing
3/4 cup pitted ripe olives, halved
5 ounces spring mix salad greens
Dash coarsely ground pepper

STEPS

1. Place the onion, garlic, celery, carrots,
   olives, cucumber, tomatoes, sweet
   peppers, salt, and pepper in a bowl;
   toss to combine.

2. Just before serving, add salad greens.
   Sprinkle with dressing and toss gently
   to combine.

3. Serve!

NUTRITION FACTS

Calories: 64 |Fat: 3 g|Carbohydrates: 7 g|Fiber: 2 g|Protein: 2 g|Sodium: 232 mg|Cholesterol: 0 mg

ASPARAGUS & CHEESE FRITTATA

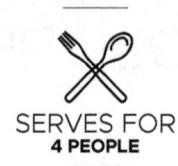

SERVES FOR
4 PEOPLE

INGREDIENTS

1/4 teaspoon salt
1/4 teaspoon pepper
1/2 cup grated Romano cheese
1/2 cup vegetable broth
1/2 cup shredded Gruyere cheese
1 medium onion, finely chopped
2 slices Italian bread (1/2 inch thick), cubed
2 tablespoons olive oil
2 cups cut fresh asparagus (1/2-inch pieces)
5 large eggs

STEPS

1. Preheat broiler. In a bowl, whisk the eggs, Romano cheese, vegetable broth, salt, and pepper until blended; stir in bread cubes.

2. In an 8-in. ovenproof skillet, heat oil over medium heat. Add onion and asparagus; cook and stir for 10 minutes.

3. Reduce heat to low; pour in egg mixture. Cook, uncovered, for 6 minutes. Sprinkle with Gruyere cheese.

4. Broil 3-4 in. from heat for 8 minutes. Let stand 5 minutes. Cut into wedges.

5. Serve!

NUTRITION FACTS

Calories: 325 |Fat: 22 g|Carbohydrates: 12 g|Fiber: 2 g|Protein: 21 g|Sodium: 779 mg|Cholesterol: 263 mg

DELICIOUS TURKEY AND MUSHROOMS

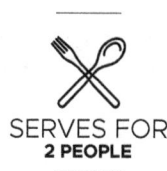

SERVES FOR
2 PEOPLE

INGREDIENTS

3/4 cup reduced-sodium beef broth
1/8 teaspoon salt
1/2 pound boneless skinless turkey
breast, cut into 2-inch strips
1 garlic clove, minced
1 tablespoon butter
1 tablespoon tomato paste
2 cups sliced fresh mushrooms

STEPS

1. In a nonstick skillet, saute garlic in butter until tender. Add turkey; cook until juices run clear. Remove and keep warm. Add the broth, tomato paste, mushrooms, and salt to skillet; cook for 5 minutes, stirring occasionally.

2. Return turkey to the pan and heat through.

3. Serve!

NUTRITION FACTS

Calories: 209 |Fat: 7 g|Carbohydrates: 5 g|Fiber: 1 g|Protein: 31 g|Sodium: 435 mg|Cholesterol: 88 mg

PORK CAESAR SALAD

INGREDIENTS

1/8 teaspoon seasoned salt
1/8 teaspoon pepper
1 tablespoon olive oil
1 tablespoon lemon juice
1 garlic clove, minced
2 tablespoons mayonnaise
SALAD:
3/4 pound pork tenderloin, cut into
1-inch cubes
1 tablespoon blackened seasoning
1 tablespoon canola oil
6 cups torn romaine
Shredded Parmesan cheese and salad
croutons

STEPS

1. For the dressing, in a bowl, mix the seasoning salt, pepper, olive oil, lemon juice, garlic, and mayonnaise until blended.

2. Toss pork with blackened seasoning. In a skillet, heat oil over medium heat. Add pork; cook and stir until tender, for 7 minutes.

3. To serve, place romaine in a bowl; add dressing and toss to coat. Garnish with pork, and croutons, and cheese.

4. Serve!

NUTRITION FACTS

Calories: 458 |Fat: 31 g|Carbohydrates: 8 g|Fiber: 3 g|Protein: 36 g|Sodium: 464 mg|Cholesterol: 100 mg

ITALIAN CLOUD EGGS

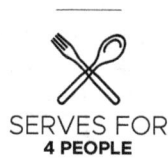

SERVES FOR
4 PEOPLE

INGREDIENTS

1/8 teaspoon salt
1/8 teaspoon pepper
1/4 teaspoon Italian seasoning
1/4 cup shredded Parmesan cheese
1 tablespoon minced fresh basil
1 tablespoon finely chopped oil-packed
sun-dried tomatoes
4 large eggs, separated

STEPS

1. Preheat oven to 450 degrees F. Separate eggs; place whites in a bowl and yolks in 4 separate small bowls. Beat egg whites, Italian seasoning, salt, and pepper until stiff peaks form.

2. In a 9-in. cast-iron skillet generously coated with cooking spray, drop egg white mixture into 4 mounds. With the back of a spoon, create a small well in the center of each mound. Sprinkle with cheese. Bake, for about 5 minutes. Gently slip an egg yolk into each of the mounds. Bake until yolks are set, for 5 minutes longer.

3. Garnish with basil and tomatoes.

4. Serve immediately.

NUTRITION FACTS

Calories: 96 |Fat: 6 g|Carbohydrates: 1 g|Fiber: 0 g|Protein: 8 g|Sodium: 234 mg|Cholesterol: 190 mg

RED PEPPER CORNMEAL SOUFFLE

INGREDIENTS

2/3 cup cornmeal
1/4 cup butter
1/2 teaspoon white pepper
1/2 teaspoon cream of tartar
1 large onion, chopped
1 teaspoon salt, divided
1 cup shredded sharp cheddar cheese
1 cup chopped sweet red pepper
2 tablespoons minced fresh parsley
2 large egg yolks, beaten
3 cups whole milk
7 large egg whites

STEPS

1. In a saucepan, saute the onion and red pepper in butter until tender. Add the milk. Bring to a boil. Gradually whisk in cornmeal; whisk constantly until thickened, about 6 minutes. Add the cheese, parsley, 1/2 teaspoon salt, and pepper. Add 1 cup cornmeal mixture to the egg yolks; mix well. Return all to saucepan.

2. In a bowl, beat egg whites, cream of tartar, and remaining salt until stiff peaks form. Fold into the cornmeal mixture. Transfer to a greased 2-qt. souffle dish.

3. Bake at 400 degrees F, for 35 minutes.

4. Serve!

NUTRITION FACTS

Calories: 193 |Fat: 11 g|Carbohydrates: 14 g|Fiber: 1 g|Protein: 9 g|Sodium: 427 mg|Cholesterol: 77 mg

VEGETABLE SCRAMBLED EGGS

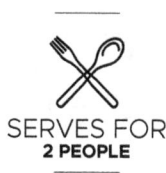

SERVES FOR
2 PEOPLE

INGREDIENTS

1/8 teaspoon pepper
1/4 cup fat-free milk
1/4 cup sliced green onions
1/4 teaspoon salt
1/2 cup chopped green pepper
1 small tomato, chopped and seeded
4 large eggs, lightly beaten

STEPS

1. In a bowl, combine the eggs and milk. Add the onions, green pepper, salt, and pepper. Pour into a lightly greased skillet. Cook and stir over medium heat until eggs are nearly set, for 3 minutes. Add tomato; cook and stir until eggs are completely set.

2. Serve!

NUTRITION FACTS

Calories: 173 |Fat: 10 g|Carbohydrates: 7 g|Fiber: 2 g|Protein: 15 g|Sodium: 455 mg|Cholesterol: 373 mg

BACON AND SWISS BREAKFAST

SERVES FOR
12 PEOPLE

INGREDIENTS

1 teaspoon seasoned salt
1 teaspoon pepper
1 pound bacon strips, cooked and crumbled
2 cups shredded Swiss cheese
2 cups 2% milk
12 large eggs
28 ounces frozen O'Brien potatoes, thawed
Minced chives

STEPS

1. In a greased 4- or 5-qt. slow cooker, bacon, layer potatoes, and cheese. In a bowl, whisk eggs, milk, seasoned salt, and pepper; pour over top.

2. Cook, covered, on low until eggs are set, for about 3 hours.

3. Turn off the slow cooker. Remove crock insert to a wire rack; let stand, uncovered, 30 minutes before serving.

4. Garnish with minced chives. Serve!

NUTRITION FACTS

Calories: 277 |Fat: 16 g|Carbohydrates: 13 g|Fiber: 2 g|Protein: 18 g|Sodium: 507 mg|Cholesterol: 220 mg

CHEESY VEGETABLE FRITTATA

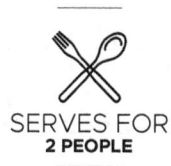

SERVES FOR
2 PEOPLE

INGREDIENTS

1/8 teaspoon salt
1/4 cup shredded sharp cheddar cheese
1/2 cup chopped fresh broccoli
1 cup sliced fresh mushrooms
2 tablespoons finely chopped onion
2 tablespoons finely chopped green pepper
2 tablespoons grated Parmesan cheese
4 large eggs, beaten
Dash pepper

STEPS

1. Preheat oven to 375 degrees F. In a bowl, combine the cheddar cheese, broccoli, mushrooms, onion, green pepper, Parmesan cheese, eggs, salt, and dash pepper. Pour into a greased shallow 2-cup baking dish.

2. Bake, uncovered, for 23 minutes.

3. Serve!

NUTRITION FACTS

Calories: 143 |Fat: 5 g|Carbohydrates: 7 g|Fiber: 1 g|Protein: 19 g|Sodium: 587 mg|Cholesterol: 14 mg

HOT FRUIT AND SAUSAGE

INGREDIENTS

3/4 cup pineapple tidbits
1 medium firm banana, sliced
2 tablespoons brown sugar
12 ounces uncooked pork sausage links
Pinch ground cinnamon

STEPS

1. In a cast-iron skillet, cook sausage according to package directions; drain.

2. Add pineapple, brown sugar, and cinnamon; heat through.

3. Stir in banana just before serving.

NUTRITION FACTS

Calories: 261 |Fat: 18 g|Carbohydrates: 14 g|Fiber: 1 g|Protein: 11 g|Sodium: 736 mg|Cholesterol: 47 mg

DILLED AND SALMON OMELETS

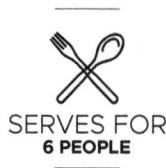

INGREDIENTS

3/4 cup sour cream
1 pound salmon fillets, cooked and flaked
2 tablespoons 2% milk
2 tablespoons butter
2 tablespoons snipped fresh dill
3 cups shredded Swiss cheese
6 fresh dill sprigs
12 large eggs
Salt and pepper to taste

STEPS

1. In a bowl, whisk the eggs, milk, salt, and pepper until blended.

2. For each omelet, in an 8-in. cast-iron skillet, melt 1 teaspoon butter over medium heat. Pour 1/2 cup egg mixture into the pan. Sprinkle with 1/3 cup salmon, 1/2 cup cheese, and 1 teaspoon snipped dill. As eggs set, lift edges, letting uncooked portion flow underneath. Cook until eggs are nearly set.

3. Broil 6 in. from the heat until eggs are completely set, for 2 minutes. Fold omelet in half; transfer to a plate.

4. Garnish with 2 tablespoons of sour cream and a dill sprig. Repeat for remaining omelets.

5. Serve!

NUTRITION FACTS

Calories: 632 |Fat: 48 g|Carbohydrates: 4 g|Fiber: 0 g|Protein: 44 g|Sodium: 374 mg|Cholesterol: 553 mg

ZIPPY BACON

INGREDIENTS

1/4 cup finely chopped pecans
1 pound bacon strips
1-1/2 teaspoons chili powder
3 tablespoons brown sugar

STEPS

1. Preheat oven to 450 degrees F. Arranges bacon in a single layer in 2 foil-lined 15x10x1-in. pan. Bake for 8 minutes; carefully pours off drippings.

2. Mix brown sugar and chili powder; sprinkle over bacon. Sprinkle with pecans. Bake until bacon is crisp, for 10 minutes. Drain on paper towels.

3. Serve!

NUTRITION FACTS

Calories: 58 |Fat: 4 g|Carbohydrates: 2 g|Fiber: 0 g|Protein: 3 g|Sodium: 151 mg|Cholesterol: 8 mg

MUSTARD HAM STRATA

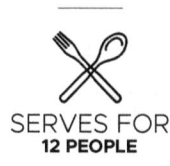

SERVES FOR
12 PEOPLE

INGREDIENTS

3/4 cup shredded cheddar cheese
3/4 cup shredded Monterey Jack cheese
1/3 cup chopped onion
1 teaspoon salt
1 cup chopped green pepper
1-1/2 cups cubed fully cooked ham
3 cups whole milk
3 teaspoons ground mustard
7 large eggs
12 slices day-old bread, crusts removed, cubed

STEPS

1. In a baking dish coated with cooking spray, layer bread cubes, ham, green pepper, onion, and cheeses. In a bowl, combine eggs, milk, mustard, and salt. Pour over top. Cover and refrigerate overnight.

2. Remove from the refrigerator 1 hour before baking. Preheat oven to 350 degrees F. Bake, uncovered, for 50 minutes. Let stand 10 minutes before cutting.

3. Serve!

NUTRITION FACTS

Calories: 198 |Fat: 11 g|Carbohydrates: 11 g|Fiber: 1 g|Protein: 13 g|Sodium: 648 mg|Cholesterol: 153 mg

CARAMELIZED BACON TWISTS

SERVES FOR
2 PEOPLE

INGREDIENTS

1/2 cup packed brown sugar
1 pound bacon strips
2 teaspoons ground cinnamon

STEPS

1. Preheat oven to 375 degrees F. Line a baking pan with foil.

2. In a bowl, mix brown sugar and cinnamon. Cut bacon strips crosswise in half; dip in sugar mixture to coat. Twist 2 times, then place in prepared pan. Bake, for 20 minutes.

3. Serve!

NUTRITION FACTS

Calories: 35 |Fat: 2 g|Carbohydrates: 3 g|Fiber: 0 g|Protein: 2 g|Sodium: 81 mg|Cholesterol: 5 mg

APPLE-SAGE SAUSAGE PATTIES

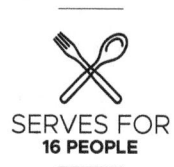

SERVES FOR
16 PEOPLE

INGREDIENTS

1/2 teaspoon pepper
1/2 teaspoon crushed red pepper flakes
1/2 cup chopped fresh parsley
1 large apple
1 large egg, lightly beaten
1-1/4 teaspoons salt
1-1/4 pounds lean ground turkey
2 garlic cloves, minced
4 tablespoons minced fresh sage
6 teaspoons olive oil, divided

STEPS

1. Peel and coarsely shred the apple; place the apple in a colander over a plate. Let stand for 10 minutes. Squeeze and blot dry with paper towels.

2. In a bowl, combine egg, parsley, sage, garlic, seasonings, and apple. Add turkey; mix lightly but thoroughly. Shape sixteen 2-in. patties. Place patties on waxed-paper-lined baking sheets. Refrigerate, covered, 8 hours.

3. In a nonstick skillet, heat 2 teaspoons oil over medium heat. In batches, cook patties for 4 minutes on each side.

4. Serve!

NUTRITION FACTS

Calories: 79 |Fat: 5 g|Carbohydrates: 2 g|Fiber: 0 g|Protein: 8 g|Sodium: 211 mg|Cholesterol: 36 mg

TOMATO-PARMESAN MINI QUICHES

INGREDIENTS

2/3 cup finely shredded Parmesan cheese
1/4 teaspoon black pepper
1/2 cup thinly sliced green onions
1 tablespoon snipped fresh basil, crushed
1 1/4 cups seeded and chopped roma tomatoes
6 eggs, lightly beaten
12 4-inch round thin slices lower sodium cooked ham
Nonstick cooking spray

STEPS

1. Preheat oven to 375 degrees F. Coat twelve 2 1/2-inch muffin cups with cooking spray.

2. Line prepared muffin cups with ham. Divide green onions, tomatoes, basil, and pepper among cups. Sprinkle with the cheese. Pour eggs over tomato mixture.

3. Bake for 20 minutes. Cool in cups for 5 minutes. Remove from cups.

4. Garnish with fresh basil.

5. Serve warm.

NUTRITION FACTS

Calories: 159 |Fat: 8 g|Carbohydrates: 5 g|Fiber: 1 g|Protein: 15 g|Sodium: 450 mg|Cholesterol: 207 mg

CHEESY AND EGG STUFFED RED PEPPERS

SERVES FOR
4 PEOPLE

INGREDIENTS

1/4 teaspoon salt
1/4 cup shredded cheese
1/4cup chopped onion
1/3 cup diced ham
1 teaspoon extra-virgin olive oil
1 tablespoon chopped fresh chives
2 large bell red peppers, plus 1/4 cup chopped, divided
2 tablespoons half-and-half
4 large eggs

STEPS

1. Preheat oven to 400 degrees F.

2. Halve 2 peppers lengthwise; remove and discard seeds. Place the peppers cut-side up in a microwave-safe dish. Microwave on High, about 4 minutes. Pat dry and sprinkle with salt.

3. Whisk eggs and half-and-half in a bowl.

4. Meanwhile, heat oil in a skillet over medium heat. Add onion and chopped bell pepper. Cook, stirring, for 3 minutes. Divide the pepper and onion mixture among the pepper halves. Divide ham among the pepper halves. Fill each pepper with the egg mixture until just filled.

5. Sprinkle each pepper half with 1 tablespoon cheese. Bake, for 30 minutes.

6. Garnish with chives and serve.

NUTRITION FACTS

Calories: 166 |Fat: 10 g|Carbohydrates: 5.5 g|Fiber: 1.4 g|Protein: 12 g|Sodium: 277 mg|Cholesterol: 206 mg

AVOCADO & SALMON OMELET

**SERVES FOR
1 PEOPLE**

INGREDIENTS

1/4 avocado, sliced
1 ounce smoked salmon
1 teaspoon extra-virgin olive oil plus 1/2 teaspoon, divided
1 tablespoon chopped fresh basil
1 teaspoon low-fat milk
2 large eggs
Pinch of salt

STEPS

1. Whisk eggs with milk and salt in a bowl.

2. Heat 1 teaspoon oil in a nonstick skillet over medium heat. Add the egg mixture and cook for about 2 minutes. Flip the omelet over and cook until set, about 40 seconds more.

3. Transfer to a plate.

4. Garnish with avocado, salmon, and basil.

5. Sprinkle with the remaining 1/2 teaspoon oil.

6. Serve!

NUTRITION FACTS

Calories: 323 |Fat: 25 g|Carbohydrates: 5 g|Fiber: 3.4 g|Protein: 19 g|Sodium: 483 mg!Cholesterol: 378 mg

CAULIFLOWER BAGEL

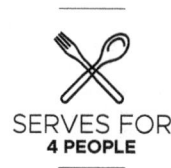

SERVES FOR
4 PEOPLE

INGREDIENTS

1 cup shredded sharp Cheddar cheese
1 large egg, lightly beaten
1 1/2 pounds cauliflower florets
2 1/2 teaspoons everything bagel
seasoning

STEPS

1. Line a baking sheet with parchment paper. Preheat oven to 425 degrees F.

2. Place cauliflower in a food processor. Process until finely chopped. Transfer to a microwave-safe bowl. Cover loosely with plastic wrap and microwave on High for 3 minutes. Let cool slightly.

3. Transfer the cauliflower to a clean kitchen towel and wring out excess moisture. Return to the bowl and stir in Cheddar and egg; mix.

4. Divide the mixture into 8 portions on the prepared baking sheet and flatten it into 3 1/2-inch circles. Using a 1-inch biscuit cutter, make a hole in the center of each circle. Remove the small circle and pat that dough onto the bagel ring. Sprinkle with seasoning.

5. Bake for 25 minutes.

6. Serve!

NUTRITION FACTS

Calories: 185 |Fat: 11 g|Carbohydrates: 8.9 g|Fiber: 3 g|Protein: 11 g|Sodium: 450 mg|Cholesterol: 75 mg

QUICK BREAD WITH SEEDED

INGREDIENTS

1/4 cup avocado oil
1/4 cup coconut flour
1/4 teaspoon salt
1/4 cup unsalted hulled sunflower seeds
1/4 cup unsalted hulled pumpkin seeds
1/2 teaspoon baking soda
1 cup buttermilk
1 tablespoon chia seeds
1 tablespoon pure maple syrup
1 tablespoon baking powder
1 3/4 cups almond flour
3 tablespoons flaxseeds
3 tablespoons sesame seeds
3 large eggs

STEPS

1. Coat a loaf pan with cooking spray. Line the bottom of the pan with parchment paper. Preheat oven to 375 degrees F. Combine the pumpkin seeds, sunflower seeds, flaxseeds, and sesame seeds in a dry skillet; toast over medium heat, stirring, for 7 minutes.

2. Reserve 2 tablespoons of the seed mixture in a bowl; transfer the remaining seeds to another bowl. Add coconut flour, almond flour, baking powder, baking soda, and salt to the large bowl; whisk to combine. Whisk eggs, oil, buttermilk, chia seeds, and maple syrup in a bowl. Stir the wet ingredients into the dry ingredients until combined. Scrape the batter into the prepared pan. Sprinkle with the reserved seeds, pressing them gently into the batter to help them adhere. Let stand for 15 minutes.

3. Bake the loaf for 40 minutes. Let cool in the pan on a wire rack for 20 minutes before turning out onto the rack to cool completely.

4. Serve!

NUTRITION FACTS

Calories: 280 |Fat: 23 g|Carbohydrates: 10 g|Fiber: 5 g|Protein: 10 g|Sodium: 349 mg|Cholesterol: 56 mg

CAULIFLOWER "TOAST"

SERVES FOR
4 PEOPLE

INGREDIENTS

1/8 teaspoon salt
1/4 teaspoon ground pepper
1 cup shredded Cheddar cheese
1 large egg, beaten
5 cups cauliflower florets
Avocado sliced

STEPS

1. Preheat to 425 degrees F. Line one large baking sheet with parchment paper. Place oven racks in upper and lower thirds of oven.

2. Place cauliflower in a food processor. Process until finely grated. Transfer to a microwave-safe bowl. Cover and microwave on High for 3 minutes. Let cool slightly.

3. Transfer the cauliflower to a clean kitchen towel and wring out excess moisture. Return to the bowl and stir in egg, Cheddar, pepper, and salt until thoroughly combined. Using about 1/4 cup of the cauliflower mixture for each, create eight 3-inch squares on the prepared baking sheet.

4. Bake for about 25 minutes.

5. Serve with sliced avocado!

NUTRITION FACTS

Calories: 166 |Fat: 11 g|Carbohydrates: 7 g|Fiber: 2.7 g|Protein: 10 g|Sodium: 315 mg|Cholesterol: 74 mg

TOFU SCRAMBLE

INGREDIENTS

3/4 cup frozen corn, thawed
1/4 cup chopped fresh cilantro
1/2 cup shredded Monterey Jack cheese
1/2 cup prepared salsa
1/2 teaspoon salt, divided
1 teaspoon ground cumin
1 small zucchini, diced
1 1/2 teaspoons chili powder
3 teaspoons canola oil, divided
4 scallions, sliced
14-ounce firm water-packed tofu, rinsed
and crumbled

STEPS

1. Heat 1 1/2 teaspoons oil in a nonstick skillet over medium heat. Add tofu, cumin, chili powder, and 1/4 teaspoon salt and cook, stirring, for about 5 minutes. Transfer to a bowl.

2. Add the remaining 1 1/2 teaspoons oil to the pan. Add the scallions, zucchini, corn, and the remaining 1/4 teaspoon salt. Cook, stirring, for 3 minutes. Return the tofu to the pan and cook, stirring, for 3 minutes more. Remove from the heat and stir in cheese until just melted. Garnish each serving with 2 tablespoons of salsa and 1 tablespoon of cilantro.

3. Serve!

NUTRITION FACTS

Calories: 202 |Fat: 12 g|Carbohydrates: 12 g|Fiber: 2.6 g|Protein: 13 g|Sodium: 508 mg|Cholesterol: 12 mg

CHICKEN WITH DRIED TOMATO CREAM SAUCE

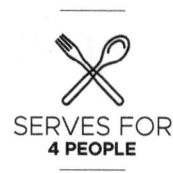

INGREDIENTS

1/4 teaspoon salt, divided
1/4 teaspoon ground pepper, divided
1/2 cup slivered oil-packed dried tomatoes, plus 1 tablespoon oil from the jar
1/2 cup finely chopped shallots
1/2 cup dry white wine
1/2 cup heavy cream
1 pound chicken cutlets
2 tablespoons chopped fresh parsley

STEPS

1. Sprinkle chicken with 1/8 teaspoon each salt and pepper. Heat dried tomato oil in a skillet over medium heat. Add the chicken and cook, turning once, until browned for about 7 minutes. Transfer to a plate.

2. Add shallots and dried tomatoes to the pan. Cook, stirring, for 2 minutes. Increase heat to high and add wine. Cook, scraping up any browned bits until the liquid has mostly evaporated, about 2 minutes. Reduce heat to medium and stir in cream, any accumulated juices from the chicken, and the remaining 1/8 teaspoon of each salt and pepper; simmer for 2 minutes. Return the chicken to the pan and turn to coat with the sauce.

3. Serve the chicken topped with the sauce and parsley.

NUTRITION FACTS

Calories: 324 |Fat: 18 g|Carbohydrates: 8 g|Fiber: 1 g|Protein: 25 g|Sodium: 249 mg|Cholesterol: 96 mg

SQUASH SOUP AND CURRY

INGREDIENTS

1/2 teaspoon garlic powder
3/4 teaspoon salt
1 medium butternut squash, peeled,
seeded and cubed
1 medium onion, chopped
2 tablespoons lime juice, plus wedges
for serving
3 cups vegetable broth
4 teaspoons curry powder
14 ounce coconut milk
Chopped fresh cilantro for garnish

STEPS

1. Stir onion, squash, broth, garlic powder, curry powder, and salt together in a 5-quart slow cooker. Cover and cook for 3 1/2 hours on High. Turn off heat and stir in coconut milk and lime juice to taste. Puree with an immersion blender until smooth.

2. Garnish with cilantro.

3. Serve!

NUTRITION FACTS

Calories: 152 |Fat: 10 g|Carbohydrates: 14 g|Fiber: 3 g|Protein: 2.2 g|Sodium: 424 mg

STUFFED PEPPERS

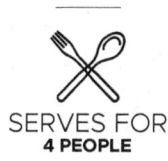

SERVES FOR
4 PEOPLE

INGREDIENTS

1/4 teaspoon salt
1/4 teaspoon ground pepper
1/4 cup chopped shallot
1/2 cup part-skim ricotta cheese
1 clove garlic, grated
2 teaspoons chopped fresh dill
2 teaspoons chopped fresh parsley
2 tablespoons extra-virgin olive oil, divided
2 red bell peppers, cut in half lengthwise and seeded
4 tablespoons shredded part-skim low-moisture mozzarella cheese, divided
6 tablespoons crumbled feta cheese
11 ounce baby spinach

STEPS

1. Preheat oven to 425 degrees F.

2. Heat 1 tablespoon oil in a nonstick pan over medium heat. Add shallot and cook, stirring often, about 1 minute. Add spinach in batches and cook, stirring, for 5 minutes. Stir garlic, dill, parsley, and pepper. Cook, stirring, for 1 minute. Transfer the spinach mixture to a mixing bowl. Stir in ricotta and feta.

3. Rub bell peppers with the remaining 1 tablespoon oil and sprinkle with salt. Divide the spinach mixture among the peppers and garnish each with 1 tablespoon mozzarella. Place in a square baking dish.

4. Bake for about 35 minutes. Let cool for 5 minutes before serving.

NUTRITION FACTS

Calories: 210 |Fat: 14 g|Carbohydrates: 11 g|Fiber: 3.4 g|Protein: 10 g|Sodium: 415 mg|Cholesterol: 26 mg

GRILLED SALMON & VEGETABLES

SERVES FOR
4 PEOPLE

INGREDIENTS

1/4 cup thinly sliced fresh basil
1/2 teaspoon salt, divided
1/2 teaspoon ground pepper
1 medium red onion, cut into 1-inch wedges
1 lemon, cut into 4 wedges
1 tablespoon extra-virgin olive oil
1 medium zucchini, halved lengthwise
1 1/4 pounds salmon fillet, cut into 4 portions
2 red bell peppers, trimmed, halved and seeded

STEPS

1. Preheat grill to medium-high.

2. Brush zucchini, peppers, and onion with oil and sprinkle with 1/4 teaspoon salt. Sprinkle salmon with pepper and the remaining 1/4 teaspoon salt.

3. Place the vegetables and the salmon pieces, skin-side down, on the grill. Cook the vegetables, turning once or twice, for 6 minutes per side. Cook the salmon, without turning, for about 10 minutes.

4. When cool enough to handle, roughly chop the vegetables and toss them together in a bowl. Remove the skin from the salmon fillets and serve alongside the vegetables. Garnish each serving with 1 tablespoon basil and serve with a lemon wedge.

NUTRITION FACTS

Calories: 281 |Fat: 12 g|Carbohydrates: 10 g|Fiber: 3 g|Protein: 30 g|Sodium: 369 mg|Cholesterol: 66 mg

LEMON-GARLIC CHICKEN

SERVES FOR
4 PEOPLE

INGREDIENTS

1/4 cup toasted pine nuts
1/4 cup unsalted chicken broth
1/4 cup dry white wine
1/2 teaspoon ground pepper, divided
1 teaspoon grated lemon zest
1 teaspoon chopped fresh thyme, plus leaves for garnish
1 tablespoon lemon juice
1 pound chicken breast cutlets
1 teaspoon salt, divided
2 tablespoons extra-virgin olive oil, divided
4 cloves garlic, thinly sliced
6 cups green beans, trimmed
Lemon wedges for garnish

STEPS

1. Sprinkle chicken with 1/2 teaspoon salt and 1/4 teaspoon pepper. Heat 1 tablespoon oil in a skillet over medium heat. Cook the chicken, turning once for 5 minutes per side. Transfer to a plate.

2. Add the remaining 1 tablespoon oil and green beans to the pan. Sprinkle with the remaining 1/2 teaspoon salt and 1/4 teaspoon pepper and cook, stirring occasionally, for about 3 minutes. Stir in garlic, lemon zest, and thyme; cook, stirring, for about 2 minutes. Add broth, wine, and lemon juice, and return the chicken and any accumulated juices to the pan. Cook, stirring occasionally until the liquid is reduced by half, about 1 minute more.

3. Serve topped with pine nuts, more thyme, and lemon wedges.

NUTRITION FACTS

Calories: 296 |Fat: 15 g|Carbohydrates: 11 g|Fiber: 3 g|Protein: 26 g|Sodium: 6525 mg|Cholesterol: 62 mg

SALMON WITH CURRIED YOGURT & CUCUMBER SALAD

INGREDIENTS

1/2 teaspoon curry powder
1/2 cup low-fat plain yogurt
1/2 teaspoon salt, divided
1/2 teaspoon ground pepper, divided
1/2 cup sliced cucumber
1 1/4 pounds sustainable wild or farmed salmon, cut into 4 portions
2 tablespoons extra-virgin olive oil, divided
2 tablespoons chopped fresh cilantro
2 tablespoons minced shallot
2 tablespoons lemon juice

STEPS

1. Brush salmon with 1 tablespoon oil and sprinkle with 1/4 teaspoon each salt and pepper. Preheat grill to medium-high.

2. Oil the grill rack. Grill the salmon, turning once for about 6 minutes.

3. Meanwhile, combine cucumber, shallot, cilantro, with the remaining 1 tablespoon oil and 1/8 teaspoon each salt and pepper in a bowl. Whisk yogurt, curry powder, lemon juice, and the remaining 1/8 teaspoon of each salt and pepper in another bowl.

4. Serve the salmon with the yogurt sauce and the cucumber salad.

NUTRITION FACTS

Calories: 258 |Fat: 12 g|Carbohydrates: 4.2 g|Fiber: 0.3 g|Protein: 30 g|Sodium: 383 mg|Cholesterol: 68 mg

SHRIMP SALAD WITH DIJON DRESSING

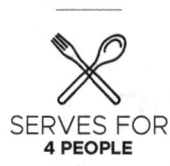

SERVES FOR
4 PEOPLE

INGREDIENTS

1/4 cup crumbled blue cheese
1/4 teaspoon salt
1/2 teaspoon ground pepper
1 avocado, diced
1 tablespoon Dijon mustard
1 cup halved cherry tomatoes
1 cup Persian cucumber chunks
2 large hard-boiled eggs, peeled and halved
2 slices cooked bacon, crumbled
2 tablespoons finely chopped shallot
3 tablespoons extra-virgin olive oil
3 tablespoons white-wine vinegar
10 cups mixed greens
12 cooked extra-large shrimp, peeled and halved lengthwise

STEPS

1. Place the oil, vinegar, mustard, shallot, pepper, and salt in a lidded jar. Shake until combined.

2. Mound salad greens on a platter. Drizzle with half the dressing and toss to coat. Decoratively arrange shrimp, cucumber, avocado, tomatoes, egg halves, bacon, and blue cheese on top.

3. Garnish with the remaining dressing. Serve!

NUTRITION FACTS

Calories: 378 |Fat: 25 g|Carbohydrates: 12 g|Fiber: 7 g|Protein: 29 g|Sodium: 516 mg|Cholesterol: 243 mg

CHICKEN, BRUSSELS SPROUTS & MUSHROOM SALAD

SERVES FOR
4 PEOPLE

INGREDIENTS

1/2 teaspoon ground pepper
1 tablespoon Dijon mustard
1 cup thinly diagonally sliced celery
1 cup shaved Parmesan cheese
1 1/2 tablespoons minced shallot
2 teaspoons chopped fresh thyme
3 tablespoons red-wine vinegar
4 cups shaved fresh cremini mushrooms
4 cups shaved Brussels sprouts
4 cups packed baby arugula
6 tablespoons olive oil
12 ounces shredded cooked chicken

STEPS

1. Whisk oil, vinegar, mustard, shallot, thyme, and pepper in a bowl. Add chicken, mushrooms, Brussels sprouts, arugula, and celery; toss to coat.

2. Garnish with Parmesan.

3. Serve!

NUTRITION FACTS

Calories: 432 |Fat: 30 g|Carbohydrates: 158 g|Fiber: 4 g|Protein: 24 g|Sodium: 532 mg|Cholesterol: 55 mg

SPANISH-STYLE CHICKEN AND CORN SOUP

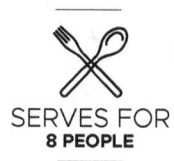

SERVES FOR
8 PEOPLE

INGREDIENTS

1/2 cup corn, fresh
1/2 teaspoon ground coriander
1/2 teaspoon salt
1 red bell pepper, seeded and chopped
1 cup lightly crushed tortilla chips, plus more for serving
1 1/2 teaspoons ground cumin
1 1/2 teaspoons crushed dried oregano
2 bay leaves
2 teaspoons lime zest
2 tablespoons lime juice
2 cups chopped onion
2 jalapeño peppers, seeded and chopped
2 cloves garlic, minced
2 pounds bone-in chicken thighs, skin removed
3 cups water
4 cups low-sodium chicken broth
15 ounce fire-roasted diced tomatoes
Diced avocado, shredded Cheddar cheese, sour cream and lime wedges for garnish

STEPS

1. Combine onion, jalapeño pepper, bell pepper, and garlic in a 5-quart slow cooker. Arrange chicken over the vegetables. Add broth, water, cumin, oregano, coriander, tomatoes, salt, and bay leaves. Cover and cook on High for 3 1/2 hours.

2. Carefully transfer the chicken to a cutting board. Shred with 2 forks.

3. Meanwhile, stir tortilla chips and corn into the slow cooker. If using the Low setting, turn to High. Cover and cook for 25 minutes more.

4. Stir the soup, breaking up any remaining pieces of tortilla chips. Stir in the chicken, lime zest, and lime juice.

5. Serve the soup with more tortilla chips, avocado, cheese, sour cream, and lime wedges.

NUTRITION FACTS

Calories: 207 |Fat: 8 g|Carbohydrates: 13 g|Fiber: 2.6 g|Protein: 20 g|Sodium: 369 mg|Cholesterol: 57 mg

HUMMUS-CRUSTED CHICKEN

INGREDIENTS

2/3 cup prepared hummus
1/4 cup toasted sesame seeds
1/4 teaspoon salt
1/2 teaspoon paprika
1/2 teaspoon ground pepper
1 teaspoon ground cumin
1 teaspoon lemon zest
2 tablespoons chopped fresh parsley
4 boneless, skinless chicken breasts
Lemon wedges for serving

STEPS

1. Line a rimmed baking sheet with foil. Preheat oven to 425 degrees F.

2. Whisk the hummus, lemon zest, cumin, paprika, salt, and pepper in a bowl. Spread the mixture evenly on both sides of chicken breasts. Sprinkle both sides with sesame seeds, pressing gently to adhere. Place on the prepared pan.

3. Roast the chicken for 25 minutes. Let stand for 5 minutes.

4. Garnish with parsley and serve with lemon wedges. Serve!

NUTRITION FACTS

Calories: 307 |Fat: 12 g|Carbohydrates: 8.7 g|Fiber: 4 g|Protein: 39 g|Sodium: 386 mg|Cholesterol: 94 mg

SEARED STEAK WITH CRISPY HERBS & ESCAROLE

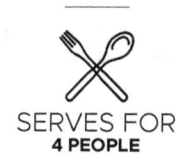

SERVES FOR
4 PEOPLE

INGREDIENTS

1/2 teaspoon salt, divided
1/2 teaspoon ground pepper, divided
1 pound sirloin steak, about 1/2 inch thick
1 sprig fresh rosemary
1 pound chopped escarole
2 tablespoons grapeseed oil or canola oil
3 sprigs fresh sage
4 cloves garlic, crushed
5 sprigs fresh thyme

STEPS

1. Sprinkle steak with 1/4 teaspoon each salt and pepper. Heat a cast-iron skillet over medium heat. Add the steak and cook on one side, for 5 minutes.

2. Turn the steak over and add oil, garlic, sage, thyme, and rosemary. Cook, stirring the herbs occasionally for 5 minutes.

3. Transfer the steak to a plate and garnish it with garlic and herbs. Tent with foil.

4. Add escarole and the remaining 1/4 teaspoon of each salt and pepper to the pan. Cook, stirring often for about 3 minutes.

5. Thinly slice the steak and serve with the escarole and crispy herbs.

NUTRITION FACTS

Calories: 244 |Fat: 11 g|Carbohydrates: 10 g|Fiber: 8.2 g|Protein: 25 g|Sodium: 393 mg|Cholesterol: 59 mg

ITALIAN CHICKEN & WHITE BEAN SOUP

INGREDIENTS

1 tablespoon chopped fresh sage, or 1/4 teaspoon dried
2 cups water
2 teaspoons extra-virgin olive oil
2 leeks, white and light green parts only, cut into 1/4-inch rounds
14-ounce reduced-sodium chicken broth
15-ounce cannellini beans, rinsed
1 2-pound roasted chicken, skin discarded, meat removed from bones and shredded

STEPS

1. Heat oil in a Dutch oven over medium heat. Add leeks and cook, stirring often, for about 4 minutes. Stir in sage and continue cooking until aromatic, about 40 seconds. Stir in broth and water, increase heat to high, cover and bring to a boil.

2. Add beans and chicken and cook, uncovered, stirring occasionally, for about 5 minutes.

3. Serve hot.

NUTRITION FACTS

Calories: 248 |Fat: 5.8 g|Carbohydrates: 14 g|Fiber: 4 g|Protein: 35 g|Sodium: 244 mg|Cholesterol: 79 mg

BAKED AVOCADO WITH SALMON & EGG

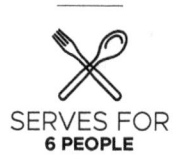

INGREDIENTS

1 tbsp chives finely chopped
3 slices smoked salmon, cut into pieces
3 large avocado
6 eggs small, separated
Pinch cayenne pepper
Toasted dark rye bread to serve

STEPS

1. Heat the oven to 400 degrees F. Halve the avocados lengthways and remove their stones.

2. Cut a small slice off the skin-side of the avocado halves to stop them rolling and put them onto a baking tray. Scoop out some of the middle from where the stone was, add a little salmon to each and then add the egg yolks.

3. Beat the egg whites quickly, so it's one uniform consistency, and pour. Grind over black pepper and bake for 12 minutes.

4. Sprinkle over the chives and a pinch of cayenne.

5. Serve with rye for dunking.

NUTRITION FACTS

Calories: 301 |Fat: 25 g|Carbohydrates: 1.8 g|Fiber: 4.5 g|Protein: 14 g|Sodium: 1.5 g

SUPERGREEN SMOOTHIE

SERVES FOR
1 PEOPLE

INGREDIENTS

1/4 cucumber, peeled and chunked
1/4 avocado, peeled and chunked
1 lime juiced
1 large kiwi fruit, juiced
Spinach handful leaves

STEPS

1. Put the spinach, cucumber, avocado,

    and fruit juices into a smoothie maker

    and whizz until smooth.

2. Serve!

NUTRITION FACTS

Calories: 139 |Fat: 7.9 g|Carbohydrates: 10 g|Fiber: 5.5 g|Protein: 3.4 g|Sodium: 0.2 g

LEMON CHICKEN WITH LEEKS AND FENNEL

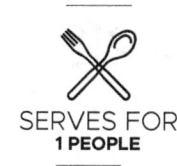

INGREDIENTS

1/2 fennel small, finely sliced
1 green beans handful
1 tbsp parsley chopped
1 tbsp tarragon finely chopped
1 lemon, juiced plus wedges to serve
1 cooked skinless chicken breast, shredded
4 baby leeks
Olive oil

STEPS

1. Whisk the 1 tsp oil, lemon juice, the tarragon, and mix well. Add the shredded chicken and leave it to marinate.

2. Heat a pan. Blanch leeks and the green beans in boiling salted water for 3 minutes, then drain. Toss the leeks and fennel slices with 1 tsp oil and season. Cook the veg in batches, and sear until charred and soft enough for a knife to go through easily. Then add to a plate with the chicken and beans.

3. Serve garnished with parsley and some lemon wedges to squeeze over.

NUTRITION FACTS

Calories: 297 |Fat: 10 g|Carbohydrates: 8.9 g|Fiber: 7.5 g|Protein: 37 g|Sodium: 0.3 g

HARISSA LAMB CUTLETS WITH TAHINI YOGURT SAUCE

SERVES FOR
PEOPLE

INGREDIENTS

1/2 tbsp clear honey
1 clove garlic, crushed
1 tbsp tahini
1 tbsp lemon juice
1 tbsp extra-virgin olive oil
1 tbsp lemon juice
2 tbsp mint leaves finely chopped
2 tbsp harissa paste
5 oz. natural yogurt
7 oz. green beans, cooked to serve
12 lamb cutlets
Sesame seeds

STEPS

1. Stir the sauce ingredients together and season. Put the chops in a dish, mix the harissa and lemon and rub them into the flesh. Leave for at least 20 minutes.

2. Heat a grill pan to high, and chargrill the chops for 3 minutes on each side, then rest. Serve the chops with the beans, a sprinkle of sesame seeds, and sauce.

NUTRITION FACTS

Calories: 462 |Fat: 28 g|Carbohydrates: 5.9 g|Fiber: 0.8 g|Protein: 46 g|Sodium: 0.5 g

CHICKEN CURRY

SERVES FOR
6 PEOPLE

INGREDIENTS

1/2 tbsp coriander
1/2 tbsp ground cumin
1/2 tbsp curry powder
1 large onion, chopped
1 tbsp ginger chopped
1 red chili, diced ground
1 small cauliflower, cut into florets
chopped
2 red peppers, seeded and diced
4 skinless chicken breasts, diced
7 oz. baby spinach
13 oz. tomatoes

STEPS

1. Blend the ginger, onion, and chili with a splash of water in a blender. Tip into a pan, and bring to a simmer. Add the spices with a pinch of salt, cook for a minute, then add the chicken, peppers, and cauliflower, stir into the curry paste and cook for another 6 minutes.

2. Add the chopped tomatoes, half-fill the tin with water, and tip into the pan. Simmer for 30 minutes. Cook for another few minutes if the sauce is too thin, then stir through the spinach until wilted.

3. Season, and serve in bowls.

NUTRITION FACTS

Calories: 170 |Fat: 2.2 g|Carbohydrates: 10 g|Fiber: 4.8 g|Protein: 24 g|Sodium: 0.7 g

STEAK WITH GARLIC MUSHROOM CREAM AND GREENS

INGREDIENTS

1 clove garlic, crushed
1 tsp Dijon mustard
2 small shallots, sliced
2 tbsp parsley chopped
2 rump steaks
3 tbsp crème fraîche
5 oz. chestnut mushrooms, finely sliced
6 oz. spinach
Olive oil
A splash chicken stock

STEPS

1. Heat 1 tbsp of olive oil in a frying pan and cook the shallot until soft. Add the garlic and cook for a minute, then add the mushrooms and cook for about 12 minutes. Stir in the crème Fraiche, mustard, and stock and bubble everything together, then stir in the parsley.

2. Brush the steaks with oil then season really well with sea salt and lots of pepper. Heat a griddle pan to high and cook the steaks for 3 minutes on each side.

3. Rest the steak for 2 minutes while you wilt the winter greens.

4. Divide between plates, garnish with a steak, and spoon over the sauce.

NUTRITION FACTS

Calories: 521 |Fat: 34 g|Carbohydrates: 5 g|Fiber: 1.9 g|Protein: 47 g|Sodium: 1.1 g

COD, CHERRY TOMATO, AND GREEN OLIVE

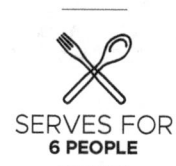

INGREDIENTS

1 red onion, cut into thin wedges
1 1/2 lb. cherry tomatoes
6 cod loin evenly sized pieces
6 parma ham pieces
18 nocellara green olives
Parsley chopped to serve
Olive oil

STEPS

1. Heat the oven to 425 degrees F.

2. Put the onions and tomatoes in a shallow roasting tin. Season, add 4 tbsp of olive oil, and toss together. Roast for 15 minutes.

3. Wrap each piece of cod in a slice of Parma ham. Add the olives to the tray and sit the cod on top of the tomatoes.

4. Keep roasting for another 15 minutes.

5. Garnish with parsley and serve!

NUTRITION FACTS

Calories: 249 |Fat: 11 g|Carbohydrates: 6 g|Fiber: 2.5 g|Protein: 28 g|Sodium: 1.4 g

VEGAN QUINOA SUSHI

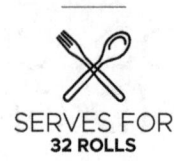

INGREDIENTS

1 tbsp maple syrup
1 tbsp rice vinegar
1 tsp maple syrup
1 tbsp mirin
1 lime, juiced
1 avocado, stoned and thinly sliced
1 carrot, peeled and shredded
1 red pepper, seeded and very thinly sliced
2 cup water
2 tbsp soy sauce
2 tbsp rice vinegar
4 nori sheets
6 oz. quinoa
A handful of leaves spinach
Teriyaki sauce
Soy sauce to serve

STEPS

1. Rinse the quinoa well, tip into a pan with water, and bring to a simmer. Cover and cook for 20 minutes. Meanwhile, mix 2 tbsp rice vinegar with maple syrup. Drain the quinoa, spread out on a plate, and leave to cool. Sprinkle over the vinegar mix.

2. To make the ponzu dipping sauce, mix all the ingredients together. To make the sushi, use a bamboo rolling mat, and cover with 1 sheet of nori. Spread some quinoa on the bottom two-thirds of the nori. Use your hands to make a 1cm thick covering. Add a layer of spinach, then the avocado, the carrot, and the peppers 1 cm up from the bottom of the quinoa. Sprinkle with the teriyaki sauce. Tightly roll the sushi from the base of the mat, to make a long thin roll. Repeat with the remaining ingredients. Chill.

3. When serving, use a wet knife to slice the sushi into 4cm lengths, serve with the soy sauce, and ginger.

NUTRITION FACTS

Calories: 35 |Fat: 1.2 g|Carbohydrates: 5 g|Fiber: 1.1 g|Protein: 1.1 g|Sodium: 0.1 g

CHOCOLATE MUG CAKE

INGREDIENTS

1/4 cup whipped cream, for serving
1/4 cup almond flour
1/2 tsp. baking powder
1 large egg, beaten
2 tbsp. butter
2 tbsp. cocoa powder
2 tbsp. chocolate chips
2 tbsp. granulated Swerve
Pinch salt

STEPS

1. Place butter in a microwave-safe mug and heat until melted, 30 seconds.

2. Add the almond flour, baking powder, egg, cocoa powder, chocolate chips, granulated Swerve, and salt, and stir until fully combined.

3. Cook for 1 minute.

4. Garnish with whipped cream to serve.

NUTRITION FACTS

Calories: 470 |Fat: 44 g|Carbohydrates: 13 g|Fiber: 7 g|Protein: 15 g|Sodium: 530 mg

MAGIC COOKIES

SERVES FOR
15 PEOPLE

INGREDIENTS

1/4 cup coconut oil
1/2 tsp. salt
3/4 cup roughly chopped walnuts
1 cup sugar-free dark chocolate chips
1 cup coconut flakes
3 tbsp. butter, softened
3 tbsp. granulated Swerve sweetener
4 large egg yolks

STEPS

1. Preheat the oven to 375 degrees F and line a baking sheet with parchment paper. In a bowl stir together butter, coconut oil, sweetener, salt, and egg yolks. Mix in coconut, chocolate chips, and walnuts.

2. Drop batter by the spoonful onto the prepared baking sheet and bake until golden, 13 minutes.

3. Serve!

NUTRITION FACTS

Calories: 130 |Fat: 13 g|Carbohydrates: 2 g|Fiber: 1 g|Protein: 2 g|Sodium: 25 mg

KETO FROSTY

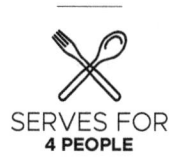

INGREDIENTS

1 tsp. pure vanilla extract
1 1/2 cup heavy whipping cream
2 tbsp. unsweetened cocoa powder
3 tbsp. keto-friendly powdered sugar
sweetener, such as Swerve
Pinch salt

STEPS

1. In a bowl, combine vanilla, cocoa, cream, sweetener, and salt. Using a hand mixer, beat the mixture until stiff peaks form. Scoop mixture into a Ziploc bag and freeze for about 30 minutes.

2. Cut the tip off a corner of the Ziploc bag and put it into the serving cups.

3. Serve!

NUTRITION FACTS

Calories: 320 |Fat: 34 g|Carbohydrates: 4 g|Fiber: 1 g|Protein: 2 g|Sodium: 35 mg

SWEET BROWNIES

INGREDIENTS

1/2 cup melted butter
1/2 tsp. salt
2 tsp. pure vanilla extract
2 tsp. baking soda
2 ripe avocados
2/3 cup keto-friendly granulated sugar
2/3 cup unsweetened cocoa powder
4 large eggs
6 tbsp. unsweetened peanut butter
Flaky sea salt

STEPS

1. Preheat oven to 350 degrees F and line a square pan with parchment paper. In a blender, combine the melted butter, salt, vanilla extract, baking soda, avocados, sugar, cocoa, eggs, and peanut butter, and blend until smooth.

2. Transfer batter to prepared baking pan and smooth top with a spatula. Garnish with flaky sea salt.

3. Bake until brownies are soft but not at all wet to the touch, for 30 minutes.

4. Let cool for 20 minutes before slicing and serving.

NUTRITION FACTS

Calories: 260 |Fat: 23 g|Carbohydrates: 11 g|Fiber: 5 g|Protein: 7 g|Sodium: 570 mg

DOUBLE CHOCOLATE MUFFINS

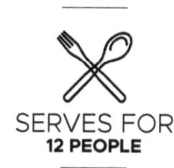

SERVES FOR
12 PEOPLE

INGREDIENTS

1/4 cup Swerve sweetener
3/4 cup unsweetened cocoa powder
1 tsp. pure vanilla extract
1 cup sugar-free dark chocolate chips
1 tsp. salt
1 cup butter, melted
1 1/2 tsp. baking powder
2 cup almond flour
3 large eggs

STEPS

1. Preheat the oven to 375 degrees F and line a muffin tin with liners. In a bowl whisk cocoa powder, almond flour, Swerve, baking powder, and salt. Add eggs, melted butter, and vanilla and stir until combined.

2. Fold in chocolate chips.

3. Divide batter between muffin liners and bake for 12 minutes.

4. Serve!

NUTRITION FACTS

Calories: 280 |Fat: 27 g|Carbohydrates: 7 g|Fiber: 4 g|Protein: 7 g|Sodium: 90 mg

COOKIE BOMBS

INGREDIENTS

1/3 cup confectioners sugar (such as Swerve)
1/2 tsp. pure vanilla extract
1/2 tsp. salt
1/2 cup butter, softened
2 cup almond flour
2/3 cup dark chocolate chip

STEPS

1. In a bowl using a hand mixer, beat butter until light and fluffy. Add the vanilla, sugar, and salt and beat until combined.

2. Slowly beat in almond flour until no dry spots remain, then fold in chocolate chips. Cover bowl with plastic wrap and place in refrigerator to firm slightly, for 30 minutes.

3. Using a cookie scoop, scoop dough into small balls.

4. Store in the refrigerator.

NUTRITION FACTS

Calories: 70 |Fat: 7 g|Carbohydrates: 2 g|Fiber: 1 g|Protein: 2 g|Sodium: 35 mg

AVOCADO POPS

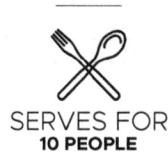

INGREDIENTS

1/3 cup juice limes
3/4 cup coconut milk
1 tbsp. coconut oil
1 cup chocolate
3 ripe avocados
3 tbsp. sugar

STEPS

1. Into a blender, combine avocados with lime juice, coconut milk, and sugar. Blend until smooth and pour into popsicle mold.

2. Freeze, for about 6 hours.

3. In a bowl, combine chocolate chips and coconut oil. Microwave until melted, then let cool to room temperature. Dunk frozen pops in chocolate and serve!

NUTRITION FACTS

Calories: 120 |Fat: 12 g|Carbohydrates: 5 g|Fiber: 3 g|Protein: 1 g|Sodium: 5 mg

CHOCOLATE TRUFFLES

SERVES FOR
15 PEOPLE

INGREDIENTS

1/4 tsp. salt
1/4 cup cocoa powder
1 cup dark chocolate chips, melted
1 medium avocado, mashed
1 tsp. vanilla extract

STEPS

1. In a bowl, combine melted chocolate, vanilla, avocado, and salt. Stir together until smooth and fully combined. Place in the refrigerator to firm up slightly, for 20 minutes.

2. When the chocolate mixture has stiffened, use a cookie scoop to scoop approximately 1 tbsp chocolate mixture. Roll chocolate in the palm of your hand until round, then roll in cocoa powder.

3. Serve!

NUTRITION FACTS

Calories: 20 |Fat: 2 g|Carbohydrates: 2 g|Fiber: 1 g|Protein: 1 g|Sodium: 35 mg

CARROT CAKE BALLS

SERVES FOR
16 PORTIONS

INGREDIENTS

1/4 tsp. ground nutmeg
1/2 tsp. pure vanilla extract
1/2 cup chopped pecans
3/4 cup coconut flour
1 block cream cheese, softened
1 tsp. stevia
1 tsp. cinnamon
1 cup grated carrots
1 cup shredded unsweetened coconut

STEPS

1. In a bowl, using a hand mixer, beat coconut flour, cream cheese, stevia, cinnamon, vanilla, and nutmeg. Fold in carrots and pecans.

2. Roll into 16 balls then roll in shredded coconut and serve.

NUTRITION FACTS

Calories: 130 |Fat: 11 g|Carbohydrates: 6 g|Fiber: 3 g|Protein: 2 g|Sodium: 65 mg

CPSIA information can be obtained
at www.ICGtesting.com
Printed in the USA
BVHW080828020621
608627BV00010B/806